Aging Families and Use of Proverbs for Values Enrichment

Aging Families and Use of Proverbs for Values Enrichment

Vera R. Jackson, DSW, ACSW
Editor

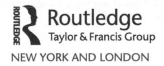

Routledge
Taylor & Francis Group

NEW YORK AND LONDON

Aging Families and Use of Proverbs for Values Enrichment has also been published as *Activities, Adaptation & Aging*, Volume 19, Number 2 1994.

The development, preparation, and publication of this work has been undertaken with great care. However, the publisher, employees, editors, and agents of The Haworth Press and all imprints of The Haworth Press, Inc., including The Haworth Medical Press and Pharmaceutical Products Press, are not responsible for any errors contained herein or for consequences that may ensue from use of materials or information contained in this work. Opinions expressed by the author(s) are not necessarily those of The Haworth Press, Inc.

First published 1994 by

The Haworth Press, Inc., 10 Alice Street, Binghamton, NY 13904-1580 USA

This edition published 2013 by Routledge
711 Third Avenue, New York, NY 10017, USA
2 Park Square, Milton Park, Abingdon, Oxfordshire OX14 4RN

First issued in paperback 2016

Routledge is an imprint of the Taylor & Francis Group, an informa business

Library of Congress Cataloging-in-Publication Data

Aging families and use of proverbs for values enrichment / Vera R. Jackson, editor.
    p. cm.
    "Aging families and use of proverbs for values enrichment has also been published as Activities, adaptation & aging, volume 19, number 2 1994"–T.p. verso
    Includes bibliographical references.
    ISBN 1-56024-725-8
    1. Aged–United States. 2. Aged–United States–Family relationships. 3. Afro-American aged.
4. Proverbs. I. Jackson, Vera R.
HQ1064.U5A6339 1995
305.26'0973–dc20   95-11389
                                                                                 CIP

ISBN 13: 978-1-138-96633-8 (pbk)
ISBN 13: 978-1-56024-725-8 (hbk)

ABOUT THE EDITOR

Vera R. Jackson, DSW, ACSW, is a Research Scientist with the George Washington University, as well as President of VEJAK Research & Management Services and Executive Director of a non-profit agency. Dr. Jackson has extensive professional experience with programs serving older persons and has developed policy intervention strategies for practitioners, administrators, educators, and researchers in the area of family proverbs transmission. She is credited with planning and implementing the first nursing home mental health component inclusive of death therapy, and has planned and implemented a "Seniors Helping Seniors" literacy program, conducted research on death, dying, and religion, and managed programs that have led to the development of intergenerational practice models. She is a member of the National Association of Social Workers and the Greater Washington Society of Association Executives.

Aging Families and Use of Proverbs for Values Enrichment

CONTENTS

PART III: HEALTH AND REHABILITATION

PART IV: LIFE EVENTS AND SPIRITUALITY

Foreword

The ways in which we perceive aging and the aged are strongly
influenced by the values of our society. These values affect our
interactions, relationships, and behaviors towards older persons and
our own responses to the aging process. In addition, these values
affect the self-concepts and actions of older persons themselves.
Although we are not always conscious of these values, they are
commonly reflected in the images of the elderly depicted in literature, in the media, and in the sayings and adages transmitted
through generations.

American society remains unclear regarding the value it places
on the aged, and indeed, on the aging process. Although much
energy and expense is devoted to increasing the life span, the value
of older people themselves remains debatable. In our youth-ori-
ented culture, aging may be perceived as good but to be old is still
of debatable worth. Rapid technological change, an emphasis on
productivity and work, have placed the value of the elderly in
jeopardy.

However, parallel to this orientation are other values which hold
age and wisdom in high esteem. Biblical edicts which demand
honor and respect for one's parents as well as underscore the counsel of the elderly continue to be upheld. The strong family ties
which persist between generations, the role that the elderly continue
to play within families, and the magnitude of assistance which
families provide to the elderly are evidence of the continued
strength of these values.

Aging involves a period of transitions and the ways in which

[Haworth co-indexing entry note]: "Foreword." Cox, Carole. Co-published simultaneously in *Activities, Adaptation & Aging* (The Haworth Press, Inc.) Vol. 19, No. 2, 1994, pp. xiii-xiv; and: *Aging
Families and Use of Proverbs for Values Enrichment* (ed: Vera R. Jackson), The Haworth Press, Inc.,
1994, pp. xiii-xiv. Multiple copies of this article/chapter may be purchased from The Haworth Document Delivery Center [1-800-3-HAWORTH; 9:00 a.m. - 5:00 p.m. (EST)].

individuals cope with these changes are strongly influenced by prevailing social values. The perceptions of chronic illnesses and the limitations they can place on activities, changes within the family, retirement, and even death itself are largely defined by our belief systems. As with other beliefs, these are often represented in expressive sayings which may dictate, either directly or indirectly, how one is to respond to these transitions.

The purpose of this volume is to examine the ways in which values, as reflected in traditional proverbs and sayings, continue to affect all aspects of the aging process. Thus, the articles explore the roles of older persons in society, within the family, and the changes which they encounter within each and within themselves. Understanding the relevance and impact of these proverbs and the ways in which they shape the aging process can increase our capacity to meet the challenge which aging presents.

Carole Cox, DSW
Associate Professor
National Catholic School of Social Service
The Catholic University of America

Acknowledgements

The editor wishes to acknowledge Patricia Villani and Phyllis Foster for their support in the conceptualization of this book. The editor also thanks her husband and children for their patience and understanding.

Finally, the editor gratefully acknowledges the contributing authors for their roles in the creation of this book. Their experience in work with older persons and their willingness to serve as proverbs guides has resulted in a book that is expected to have a significant impact upon older persons and their proverbs henceforth.

Introduction

Service delivery to older persons has moved towards a value based approach emphasizing the importance of an individual's belief structure. Moreover, respect for diversity has prompted practitioners to consider the variability of older persons in regards to proverbs, beliefs, values and behaviors.

The intent of this book is to examine human competencies, coping mechanisms, and limitations within a proverbs context. This book is based upon best practices in the use of proverbs as transmitters of values and as assessment tools. This book also offers information and insights from contributing authors who have professional and personal experiences with the use of proverbs.

The major objective of this book is to present administrators, practitioners, educators, researchers, and students with intervention models that acknowledge and build upon the proverbs orientation of the client. This objective guides the underlying philosophy that those providing services to older persons must develop intervention strategies that are relevant to older persons.

This work is organized into four parts with headings labeled according to topical categories to facilitate the reader's identification of areas of interest. Part I is an effort by the editor to provide the reader with a framework for understanding proverbs and their relationship to values.

Part II introduces the reader to the intergenerational transmission of proverbs. Suggestions are provided to help practitioners work

[Haworth co-indexing entry note]: "Introduction." Jackson, Vera R. Co-published simultaneously in *Activities, Adaptation & Aging* (The Haworth Press, Inc.) Vol. 19, No. 2, 1994, pp. 1-2; and: *Aging Families and Use of Proverbs for Values Enrichment* (ed: Vera R. Jackson) The Haworth Press, Inc., 1994, pp. 1-2. Multiple copies of this article/chapter may be purchased from The Haworth Document Delivery Center [1-800-3-HAWORTH; 9:00 a.m. - 5:00 p.m. (EST)].

more effectively with older persons within the confines of their cultural, ethnic, and familial experiences.

Part III illustrates proverbs' influence upon health and restorative services considered by older persons. Implications and strategies for work with older persons are outlined as the reader is led through the intervention process.

Part IV offers an insight into proverbs as a buffer for stress, change, loss, and many other challenges confronting older persons. The contributions in this section serve as an opportunity to enhance the sensitivity and awareness of interventionists to the link between proverbs and spirituality.

Vera R. Jackson, DSW, ACSW

PART I

THE PROVERBS FRAMEWORK

Chapter 1

Proverbs:
A Tool for Work with Older Persons

Vera R. Jackson

SUMMARY. Proverbs are regarded as a resource for both understanding and providing services to older persons. Examples of proverbs are cited and exchange theory is offered as a framework for considering the proverbs transmission process. The discussion concludes with a model for developing a proverbs assessment and intervention plan.

Many elderly persons convey, within the context of the helping relationship, value statements commonly known as proverbs, that may positively or negatively dictate self-acquisition or self-maintenance practices related to good physical health, psychosocial well-being or overall quality of life. Correspondingly, many practitioners

Vera R. Jackson, DSW, ACSW, is President of VEJAK Research & Management Services, Executive Director of a non-profit agency, and Research Scientist with the George Washington University. Dr. Jackson received a BA in Psychology and Sociology from Trinity College and a MSW and DSW with a specialty in gerontology from Howard University. She is a member of the National Association of Social Workers and the Greater Washington Society of Association Executives, in addition to maintaining membership on several boards and civic organizations.

Address correspondence to: 5808 Westbrook Drive, New Carrollton, MD 20784.

[Haworth co-indexing entry note]: "Proverbs: A Tool for Work with Older Persons." Jackson, Vera R. Co-published simultaneously in *Activities, Adaptation & Aging* (The Haworth Press, Inc.) Vol. 19, No. 2, 1994, pp. 5-13; and: *Aging Families and Use of Proverbs for Values Enrichment* (ed: Vera R. Jackson) The Haworth Press, Inc., 1994, pp. 5-13. Multiple copies of this article/chapter may be purchased from The Haworth Document Delivery Center [1-800-3-HAWORTH; 9:00 a.m. - 5:00 p.m. (EST)].

have acknowledged that proverbs influence interaction, but have as yet to regard proverbs as an intervention tool.

This paper offers a perspective of proverbs as a critical element of the decision-making process of older persons and as an equally critical and viable resource to practitioners. The discussion begins with an exploration of proverbs, their relationship to values, and their transmission. At the conclusion of this discussion, a model is offered for the development of a proverbs assessment and intervention tool.

FAMILY PROVERBS

Family proverbs are adages, stories (Stone, 1988; Page & Washington, 1987), words of wisdom (Pasteur & Toldson, 1982) or religious instruction reflecting a family's attitudinal or belief structure. Proverbs provide images of physical, psychological, emotional and spiritual beliefs. Often poetic, prosaic and emotionally powerful, they allow for free expression with a natural rhythm. They have a meaning and simplicity that transcends words, but are understood by the speaker. Proverbs shape lives—consider the proverb, "an apple doesn't fall too far from the tree."

Through the sharing of proverbs, family members provide strategies for self-preservation, influence decisions and judgments (Pasteur & Toldson, 1982), affect educational, career, or marital pursuits (Stone, 1988; Page & Washington, 1987) and transmit values from generation to generation (McAdoo, 1989; Page & Washington, 1987). Within some families, proverbs and values are so interrelated that they are considered as one in the same. This discussion will treat proverbs from the aforementioned perspective, as a value, having both guiding and directing impacts upon thoughts and behavior.

Throughout the life course, proverbs are differentially reinforced by society, significant others, and reference groups (Fine, Schwebel, James-Myers, 1987). Families are most often the conduits or "transmitters" of proverbs. Family proverbs may either agree or disagree with societal values. Proverbs are also garnered through relationships in cultural, ethnic, racial, socioeconomic, educational, and religious groupings. Moreover, proverbs sharing often occurs within fraternal and service organizations, health, education, and welfare institutions, political groups, and neighborhoods.

Proverbs are often as diverse as the people who believe them. They have managed to become a central thread in the fabric that guides thoughts and behaviors. Proverbs often have a far reaching impact upon the general well being and quality of life of those who have been exposed to them. For this reason, one must consider the proverbs transmission process and implications for intervention.

PROVERBS TRANSMISSION

Exchange theory offers an appropriate framework for considering the decision-making process related to the transmission of proverbs. The general proposition of exchange theory is that humans avoid costly behavior and seek rewarding status, relationships, and interaction to the end that their profits are maximized. According to Nye (1982), there are five major components of exchange theory: (1) rewards–the physical, psychological and social spheres of an individual's life; (2) costs–any status, relationship, interaction, milieu, or feelings disliked by the individual; (3) profits/benefits– the outcome that provides the best relationship of rewards to costs; (4) comparison level–the standard by which individuals evaluate the rewards and costs of a relationship in terms of what they feel they deserve from that relationship; and, (5) norm of reciprocity– people help those who help them.

Social exchange involves actions that create diffuse future obligations. It involves making investments that constitute some level of commitment or obligation to the other party. In this context, proverbs are shared because they have special meaning to family members, there is a mutual trust between family members that the process will not be lost, and a reward system (either internal or external) is linked with the transmission.

Exchange theory suggests that families will continue to do what they found rewarding in the past. If an individual adopts a belief in a proverb, and receives a certain amount of pleasure (healthy or unhealthy) that individual will be more inclined to share the proverb with other family members. Moreover, once there is family acceptance of a proverb, families are less likely to consider other proverbs outside of those they already believe in.

The family proverbs transmission ritual is acted out in a systematic fashion over time contributing significantly to the establishment and preservation of a sense of self. This ritual allows for the establishment of boundaries, stabilizes the family, and promotes identity formation.

Families who pay close attention to the past, whether they refer to prior generations or to events of the previous year, are more likely to preserve the family proverbs transmission. For them, ritualistic activity related to the sharing of proverbs is consciously planned and taught to other family members.

Examples

Proverbs touch upon all facets of life and may encompass many different spheres of existence, including but not limited to the physical, psychological, emotional, developmental and spiritual. It is virtually impossible to fully grasp the intrinsic worth of proverbs to older persons without considering a few diverse examples.

Proverbs often used to refer to mental, emotional, developmental or physical differences

1. You can't teach an old dog new tricks.
2. You can lead a horse to water but you can't make him drink.
3. There may be snow on the roof but there's fire in the furnace.
4. Age before beauty.
5. Age is but a number.
6. You're as young as you feel.
7. With the ancient is wisdom; and in length of days understanding.
8. The race is not won by the swiftest, but he who endures to the end.
9. Youth is wasted on the young.

Proverbs often used to refer to self-help, health and prevention

10. An apple a day keeps the doctor away.
11. Early to bed, early to rise makes a man healthy, wealthy, and wise.
12. An ounce of prevention is worth a pound of cure.
13. You are what you eat.

Proverbs often used to refer to a desire for a lack of knowledge

    14. No news is good news.
    15. What you don't know can't hurt you.

Proverbs often used to refer to periods of time

    16. There's no time like the present.
    17. There's always tomorrow.
    18. This is a new day.
    19. Today is the first day of the rest of your life.
    20. For everything there is a season.

Proverbs often used to denote hope and expectations

    21. Hope springs eternal.
    22. Trouble don't last always.
    23. Every dark cloud has a silver lining.
    24. Its always darkest before the dawn.

Proverbs often used to refer to learned life experiences

    25. Some people you meet on the way up, you'll meet on the way down.
    26. Don't burn your bridges.
    27. Everything that glitters isn't gold.
    28. The grass is always greener on the other side.
    29. Don't put all your eggs in one basket.
    30. Every house is not a home.

Proverbs considered to have religious or spiritual implications

    31. God loves the hoary hair.
    32. Train up a child in the way he should go; and when he is old, he will not depart from it.

ASSESSMENT AND INTERVENTION

Proverbs are an appropriate tool for work with older persons on both an individual and a group basis. As mentioned earlier, this mode of communication is based upon verbal input and output. The process of proverbs sharing in large part is influenced by the individual's past experiences.

With Individuals

On an individual level, proverbs yield the opportunity of looking at older persons (and individual family members) in terms of: (1) the proverbs that are specific to the culture they represent; (2) the proverbs that they are operating from; and, (3) the proverbs that may be in conflict with the helping relationship. This proverb assessment data may lead to the development of early intervention, individual counseling, and late life planning of older persons relative to their psychosocial functioning.

Interventionists must consider a paradigm of ethnic competence in the assessment that includes proverbs clarification by the interventionist, collection and analysis of information regarding the individual's cultural family and an examination of the individual's agreement (as well as the family's) with or "belief in" specific proverbs. Using this model will help to ensure that the assessment is focused upon the older person and is relevant to cultural and familial experiences.

The following steps should be considered in the assessment and intervention process.

1. Compile a list of proverbs.

Organize focus groups with a representative sample of clients, families, and service providers. Ask the groups to brainstorm a list of proverbs and to attach a meaning to each proverb. Should the group experience difficulty in determining a meaning for each proverb, try to agree to no more than two strong possible meanings for each proverb.

2. Through client interviews (and where possible family member interviews), determine the belief structure.

Ask the client which proverbs they were taught by family members. Determine which proverbs they believe, why, and what meaning is associated with them. If the client is unable to convey a meaning for a proverb, utilize the information garnered from your focus groups as probes.

3. After reviewing this data, determine whether proverbs are in concert with or a hindrance to service delivery.

This exploration should offer a perspective of the proverbs associated with a belief that may impact your intervention with a client. If a proverb is viewed as a benefit to the helping relationship, make references to that proverb throughout the helping process. If a proverb is viewed as a hindrance to the health and welfare of the client, convey proverbs previously identified that offer a more positive perspective. For example, an older person who believes "what you don't know can't hurt you" may be more prone to seek critical medical care if this proverb is countered with a proverb suggesting empowerment like, "an ounce of prevention is worth a pound of cure." Similarly, an older person who believes, "you can't teach an old dog new tricks," may be receptive to restorative services if this proverb is offset by one suggesting self-worth and insight like, "with the ancient is wisdom; and in length of days understanding."

With Groups

A proverbs assessment tool also offers a framework for understanding group (or family), organizational dynamics and composition. At this level, individual proverbs are assessed and reviewed in relationship to the group's beliefs. This tool provides a sound foundation for the identification and development of supportive measures to allow groups to maintain cohesiveness and direction. Practitioners may address issues relevant to the their respective fields while focusing upon the implication for cultural learning.

Projections that people of color will populate over one third of the nation have implications for pluralistic human services delivery. For example, proverbs may be used by human service organizations to conduct program evaluations and to determine strengths and weaknesses. This tool may also serve as the basis for cross cultural training designed to dispel myths and stereotypes, as well as unveil organizational attitudes that interfere with the full contributions of older persons who have remained an active part of the work force.

The following model serves as a framework for the application of proverbs as an assessment tool with groups and organizations.

There are many similarities between this model and that of the model for use with individuals.

1. Compile a list of proverbs.

When working with groups and organizations, a focus group of representatives from these entities will serve as a catalyst for determining their cultural proverb system. Ask the groups to brainstorm a list of proverbs and to attach a meaning to each proverb. Should the group have difficulty in determining a meaning for each proverb, try to agree to no more than two strong possible meanings.

2. Determine the belief structure.

Ask group members to indicate their agreement with each proverb. This task can be accomplished by simply asking them to score each proverb from 1 to 10; 10 = strong agreement with the truth in the proverb 1 = strong disagreement with the truth in the proverb.

3. Analyze and discuss the responses with the group.

Tally the responses for each proverb and engage the group in discussions of the implications for agreement and disagreement.

4. Strategize and implement ways of utilizing proverbs as a means for encouraging group cohesiveness and diversity.

Administrators interested in creating work environments that deemphasize age differences and negate stereotypes about older workers should consider integrating proverbs into their human resource development plans. For example, training curricula can include a discussion of proverbs that promote staff unity regardless of age differences like, "age is but a number" and "you're as young as you feel."

Therapists and other practitioners engaged in family or group work may also utilize proverbs as a vehicle for breaking down barriers and resolving conflicts. Stereotypical references to aging and older persons may be countered by proverbs that address positive images of older persons and their contributions like, "God loves the hoary hair" and "with the ancient is wisdom; and in length of days understanding."

CONCLUSION

Proverbs are relevant to all helping strategies for older persons. They serve as a catalyst for work with individuals, families, and groups and offer empowerment opportunities for older persons and their service providers.

Proverbs have been presented as being causally linked to older persons' social and personal identities including subsequent behaviors. The challenge now rests with service providers, regardless of discipline, to set the standard for integrating proverbs into intervention plans for the benefit and well being of all older persons.

AUTHOR NOTE

Dr. Jackson has developed policy and intervention strategies for practitioners, educators, and researchers in the area of family proverbs transmission. In addition, she has conducted research and written articles and manuals on depression and aging, mental health planning in nursing homes, religiosity and spirituality, rehabilitation, chronic illness and death and dying.

REFERENCES

Fine, M., Schwebel, A.I., James-Myers, L. (1987, Spring). Family stability in black families: Values underlying three different perspectives. *Journal of Comparative Family Studies*, 28, (1), 1-23.

King James Version, *Bible*.

McAdoo, H.P. (1989, November, 10). Family values and outcomes for children. Paper presented at the One-Third of a Nation; African American Perspectives Conference. Washington, D.C.: Howard University.

Nye, F. I. (1982). *Family relationships: Rewards and costs*. Beverly Hills: Sage Publications.

Page, M. & Washington, N. (1987). Family proverbs and value transmission of single black mothers. *Journal of Social Psychology*, 127, (1), 49-58.

Pasteur, A.B. & Toldson, I.L. (1982). *Roots of Soul: The Psychology of Black Expressiveness*. Garden City, New York: Anchor Press/Doubleday.

Stone, E. (1988,April). How family stories shape us. *Glamour*, 290-320.

PART II

CULTURE AND FAMILY

Chapter 2

A Cultural Exchange of Values

Pamela L. McKee

SUMMARY. The aged in various cultures assume the responsibility to teach values to each generation within the family. In most instances, these values are taught through stories and proverbs that are handed down from one generation to another and become the cornerstone of life lessons for members of that family. "Don't make your eye long behind anything you see anyone has, since you do not know if they hold the Devil by his tail to get it and you may not want to pay the same price," was one of the proverbs shared by my grandmother, great-aunts, aunts and mother to ensure that one was not jealous or envious of material things owned by others.

A CULTURAL EXCHANGE OF VALUES

Early childhood in the West Indies was an exciting time during the fifties. During this period, my two brothers, two sisters and I enjoyed an extended family that included aunts and uncles not only residing in Trinidad and Tobago but also in Grenada. When our great-aunts (one on our mother's side and the other on our father's side–as must be firmly declared when referring to relatives in the

---

Pamela L. McKee holds a BS degree in Psychology and an MA in Education Administration from Howard University.

Address correspondence to: 431 Oneida Place, N.W., Washington, DC 20011.

[Haworth co-indexing entry note]: "A Cultural Exchange of Values." McKee, Pamela L. Co-published simultaneously in *Activities, Adaptation & Aging* (The Haworth Press, Inc.) Vol. 19, No. 2, 1994, pp. 17-26; and: *Aging Families and Use of Proverbs for Values Enrichment* (ed: Vera R. Jackson) The Haworth Press, Inc., 1994, pp. 17-26. Multiple copies of this article/chapter may be purchased from The Haworth Document Delivery Center [1-800-3-HAWORTH; 9:00 a.m. - 5:00 p.m. (EST)].

Caribbean) and grandmother (on our father's side, since I was too young to remember my maternal grandmother's jaunt to see us) came to visit, you would have thought we were expecting the Queen of England.

Our uncles and aunts were received with similar, though not equal, pomp and circumstance and, therefore, did not generate the same levels of enthusiasm. We suspected that they had not yet earned the homage paid to the aged in our culture during that period since they were only one generation above us in rank.

The West Indies is a chain of islands bordered by the Atlantic Ocean to the east, the Caribbean Sea to the north, the Gulf of Paria to the west and the Columbus Channel to the south. The island, formerly inhabited by the Arawak and Carib Indians, was ruled by the Spanish, French, Dutch and British over its many years of colonization before it gained independence from the British on August 31, 1962 (Trinidad and Tobago Statistical Pocket Digest, 1983).

The history of the growth of the island's population began when the Spanish king issued his first decree in 1777, followed by another in 1783, inviting the French from Haiti, Martinique, St. Lucia and other islands then colonized by the French, to come to Trinidad and take up residence. One criterion was stipulated within those decrees: that the invitees must be of the Roman Catholic faith (Ottley, 1972). In its development and ensuing history, its annual carnival, which was originally introduced by French settlers who came to the island in the late eighteenth century (Ahye, 1983), calypso music and its distinction as "the birthplace of the steelband" (Goddard, 1991) played a significant role in the pattern of migration.

Today, the country is home to approximately 1.3 million inhabitants represented by Black, East Indian, White, Chinese, Mixed and "Other" ethnic groups with its language flavored predominantly by inflections from the British and seasoned by accents from each of the smaller West Indian islands. The rhythmic pattern of speech and potpourri of phrases sprinkled during conversations attest to the pattern of easy flow and interconnectedness among the inhabitants of the various islands and migration from the north to the southernmost tropical island.

Trinidad and Tobago is described as a country "rich in its cultural heritage–with contributions made by more than a score of different races–a veritable treasure house of vari-colored gems to which each race–the Amerindians, the French and Spanish settlers, the Negro slaves, the English, East Indians (Hindu, Mohammedan and others), the Chinese, Portuguese, and Syrians have contributed" (Ahye, 1983). The history of the country dates the importation of the Amerindians, during the period of Spanish colonialism, from the South American continent to work the then-booming sugar plantation and the thriving tobacco fields of that era (Williams, 1962).

The island is best known for its exports of oil, sugar, citrus, and cocoa and carries the banner of host to the greatest show on earth: its carnival and steelband music. The steelband is credited with playing a significant role " as a great instrument of social control" in the lives of young men (Frost, 1975).

My mother and father emigrated from Grenada to Trinidad and Tobago, West Indies during their early adult lives. Brothers and sisters followed immediately after, and this pattern offered an immediate nucleus of aunts and uncles, many of whom lived in close proximity to each other. The cousins of this generation were not prepared to be left behind and some followed to join the group, care for each other's children, give unsolicited but appreciated advice and, over the many years, serve as godmothers and godfathers to the newborns.

While the babies from each family were introduced to relatives with controlled enthusiasm and pride, the older members were displayed as the "pearls" of the family–they knew who and what they were and we understood this at a very early age.

Family activities during those times were very basic. We buzzed around keeping the yard clean with brooms made from the spine of coconut branches, concocted special drinks and made deserts, especially ice cream, from various fruits including soursop, barbadine, and coconut milk. As children we played a special role in our mode of communication as we announced to relatives, friends and neighbors that "Auntie" or "Tantie" or "MaMa" was expected to pay us a visit and "spend time with us" within the next several weeks or months.

Travel plans were made very early since the delivery of mail from one island to another was dependent on the boats which visited the chain of islands each week and our technical environment did not lend itself to the immediate use of a telephone (there were usually one or two phones per street in our neighborhood). In many instances, the fact that one had access to a telephone on one island did not guarantee access by your relative on another island.

During this period of our country's development, we depended on face-to-face visits and the most amazing super information highway that involved taking the word to relatives and friends in one particular neighborhood and being assured that the "message" will be passed on to the others in the "network." The information was delivered without fail on each occasion.

The anticipation on our end was not in vain. We were rewarded with special homemade treats as we watched our parents receive their fantasized foods and fruits peculiar to the land they left many years ago. Since these visits lasted a minimum of one to three months, they gave our parents an opportunity to reminisce about their childhoods, catch up on the latest update from their neighborhoods and to hear once again, the stories they heard over and over from their aunts, uncles and parents when they were children.

It was our "Aunt Brick" who told the most stories during her visits. It was at her knees I first learned the proverb: "Don't make your eyes long behind anything you see anyone has, you do not know if they hold the Devil by his tail to get it and you may have to pay the same price for it."

The internal tape on which this proverb is recorded has played itself over and over in my psyche during the several decades of my life each time I hear someone become excited about something owned or received by someone else and express the desire (sometimes to the level of obsession) to have the same or similar item. It was the most declarative life-lesson I learned to ensure that I would not be envious or jealous of my friends or wish to have anything they possessed.

The fabric of the proverb was usually interwoven in a story of love between a male and female and the desire of another female or male for the same man or woman. Sometimes it varied with reflections on material possessions one gained through hard work, sacrifice or "strange practices." The latter framework for these stories would leave us scared to close the windows or complete any other assigned task once it became dark. During the night, our young minds would play the stories over and over again with the tape sometimes becoming stuck on the proverb.

Over the years, it was interesting to hear my mother and father repeat this proverb to us as we grew into our teenage years and began to develop friendships with special individuals in school. As part of our socialization process into adulthood, one of these individuals is usually promoted to "best-friend" status and it is this friend who serves as the catalyst for the most distinct and vivid memories of experiences outside of the home and the worse memories of family conflict on the inside. Each average childhood brings with it these conflicts, and my special conflict came during the Easter holiday.

In the Caribbean, Easter is a very special time of renewal and celebration second only to Christmas. In Trinidad and Tobago a significant percentage of the population are Roman Catholics who participate in the rituals of the celebration of this season which is preceded by Lent–a period of abstinence from certain activities, including dancing. Over the years, the restrictions have waned but during this period, Easter marked a very special occasion in the life of a pre-adolescent female.

Easter Sunday excursions were planned to various parts of the country. Many of these family activities involved travelling several miles by train to visit other churches, travelling several hours by boat to visit smaller islands where we would disembark and spend the day swimming, eating and visiting the sites the island had to offer, or travelling by car to beaches for an all-day picnic of grand meals to be shared among other attendees, relatives and friends.

The preparations for these excursions began on Saturday, continued with boarding your mode of transportation for your travels very early the next morning and culminated on Sunday evening with a team that was exhausted by our walk to the church site after leaving the train station, the blast of the ocean waves against our bodies, or from eating too much of the meals made and shared by an aunt or your parents' good friends.

As we made plans for one special Easter outing during my last year in elementary school, I visited my good girlfriend and her sisters and joined them on a trip to their seamstress to be fitted for their Easter dresses. During this period in the Caribbean, clothing was not purchased "off the rack." Each family had its at-home resident seamstress in the mother or big sister or a seamstress in its immediate neighborhood. In a few instances one would have a seamstress in another area which involved travelling by bus or car to be measured for the clothing of one's choice after purchasing the material and deciding on the design (yes, there were budding designers at early ages) or the choice of style as depicted in the most current fashion magazines.

My mother and older sister were the resident seamstresses in our household for me, the youngest female in the family. Their clothing, together with that of my second sister's, was sewn by a seamstress in the neighborhood. I guess I had not yet graduated to having my clothing sewn by the "neighborhood seamstress" since I was not a wage earner.

The comradery shared with my friend and her sisters was probably the significant contributor to my independent spirit upon my return home, when I approached my mother to discuss the dress my girlfriend tried on and requested to have my Easter dress made by the same woman. My breathless description of the details of color, style and grand fitting was greeted with my mother launching into a tirade that would last a full two weeks during which I was constantly reminded of my great-aunt's proverb, which now belonged to my mother by virtue of her maturity and stature as the next senior generation and by my greataunt's absence. She prefaced her scolding with full copyright credit to all of the ancestors on her side of the family as well as to those on my father's side of the family as she stood before me with her hands on hips with full authority: "Old people say, don't make your eyes long behind anything you see anyone have. You don't know if they hold the Devil by his tail to get it, you don't know what your friend and her mother do to get that dress and you may have to pay the same price for it." In one quick moment of madness I took leave of my senses and it took one quick moment of repetition to restore my sanity.

Today, psychologists may dissect this proverb repeated in the context of this story and debate whether my mother and all of her female relatives came from a dysfunctional family which left her in a state of emotional and material deprivation to elicit such a reaction. Attorneys may dissect this proverb repeated in this context and find cause for a suit against my mother, grandmother and great-aunts for defamation of character or slander. In the latter instance, however, I would step forward unhesitatingly and serve as the principal witness in defense of my relatives as I have heard myself repeat this proverb to my nieces, nephews, great-niece and friends over many years.

The activities of the aged in the Caribbean are not studied and delivered in the same formal setting as is done here in the United States. In this culture, there exists an array of social services in community-based multipurpose and nutrition centers that are supported and fueled by the Older Americans Act, through the State Agencies on Aging. These multipurpose centers offer a variety of activities which include, among other areas of focus, literacy training, health promotion, counseling, recreation and socialization, transportation, home-delivered meals, telephone reassurance and other support systems for the elderly designed to keep the elderly active in their communities.

On the other hand, the emphasis in other cultures seeks to maintain the status of these adults among their family members and within a community where the older adults are revered and depended upon to play certain roles within the immediate family. Oftentimes, this role and the contributions offered continue outside of the immediate family into the broader community or neighborhood which, in the absence of immediate family members or significant others, assumes direct responsibility for its elders.

The editors of *Psychology and the Older Adult: Challenges for Training in the 1980s, "Status and Role Shifts,"* cite research which indicate that the social changes accompanying the later years can be summarized in one word—loss. Reference is made to a study completed by Rosow (1973, 1976) which articulates the following five aspects of role loss in old age:

1. The loss of roles excluded elderly persons from significant social participation and devalues them;

2. Old age is the first stage of life in which there is systematic status loss for an entire cohort;
3. Individuals are not socialized to the fate of aging (i.e., role losses are institutionalized but socialization to them is not);
4. The elderly tend to live socially unstructured lives because society does not specify an aged role; and
5. Role loss deprives elderly persons of their social identity.

The elderly, according to this study, are portrayed as experiencing severe discontinuity, increased social ambiguity, few formal rites of status passage, and loss of instrumental value. The impact of these combined forces are described as a "process [that] steadily eats away at these crucial elements of social personality . . . a direct, sustained attack on the ego . . . which deprives them of their very social identity" (Rosow, 1976).

The roles of the older adults (grandparents, great-aunts, and great-uncles, uncles and aunts) during that period of my early childhood and in the lives of my friends and schoolmates were very defined, structured and designed to maintain continuity of their status as statespersons within the family. They were the roving story-telling ambassadors of our generation who taught and reinforced the values of the family through their annual visits which were heralded by simple hand-made delicacies and stories told to the children of their daughters and sons, or nieces and nephews.

They brought with them a tenderness and acceptance of our youth and allowed us to share with them our tenderness and acceptance of their aging. We laughed, sang songs and listened far into the night to their stories, each of which contained a proverb. These proverbs will be repeated to us over and over upon each visit and reinforced by our mothers, fathers, aunts and uncles during their absence.

It has served as the agent of the value lesson taught to declare me free of envying anything owned or received by any good friend (or not so good friend) or contemporaries. It is the one proverb I packed with me when I travelled from the Caribbean to take up residence in the United States, where I have lived for approximately twenty-five years.

This proverb has been shared with friends who know it very well, understand its meaning and the valuable lessons taught by its repetition from one generation to the other. It binds me to my grandmother, great-aunts, aunts and uncles to the same degree that it now serves as the thread that weaves special friendships and shared values in another country thousands of miles away from Grenada and Trinidad and Tobago. My friends have laughingly repeated it back to me over the years and, I am sure, they have repeated it to their children, nieces, nephews and great-nieces.

My hope is that it is also repeated and will continue to be repeated to their grandchildren in the years ahead.

AUTHOR NOTE

The author is affiliated with Alumni of Leadership Washington, Class of 1994; Board Member, District of Columbia Chamber of Commerce; Board Member, Casa Iris; Member, Women of Washington; Member, National Association of Female Executives. Since moving to the United States in 1969, she has served in various capacities including Special Assistant for Administration during the Carter Administration, President and Manager of her own retail business for six years and Executive Director of a large Social Service agency. Recently, she ventured out on her own again as a Program Development Consultant using her experience in aging, mental health, economic development and youth services to serve both public and private organizations.

The author thanks her grandmothers, great-aunts, aunts, uncles, brothers, sisters, nieces, nephews and great-niece and most of all her parents Thomas and Claire McKee. Special thanks to Michael, Joan and Alexa Dupigny for the resources they made available.

REFERENCES

Ahye, Molly, *Cradle of Caribbean Dance: Beryl McBurnie and the Little Carib Theatre*. Republic of Trinidad and Tobago: Heritage Cultures Ltd., 1983.

Frost, David, *David Frost Introduces Trinidad and Tobago*. Michael Anthony and Andrew Carr (Eds.), London: Andre Deutsch Limited, 1975.

Goddard, George "Sonny," *Forty Years in the Steelbands 1939-1979*. Roy D. Thomas (Ed.), Republic of Trinidad and Tobago: Karia Press, 1991.

"Trinidad and Tobago Statistical Pocket Digest," prepared by the Ministry of Finance, Central Statistical Office, 1985.

Ottley, C. R., *The Story of Trinidad and Tobago in a Nutshell.* Port-of-Spain: Horsford Printerie, 1972.

Rosow, I., The Social Context of Aging. *Gerontologist,* 1973, 13, 82-87.

Rosow, I., R. Binstock and E. Shanas, (Eds.) Status and Role Change Through the Life-Span. *Handbook of Aging and the Social Sciences.* New York: Van Nostrand Reinhold, 1976.

Santos, John F. and Gary R. VandenBos, (Eds.), Psychology and the Older Adult: Challenges for Training in the 1980s. Washington, D.C.: American Psychological Association, Inc., 1982.

Williams, Eric, *History of the People of Trinidad and Tobago.* Port-of-Spain, Trinidad, W.I.: PNM Publishing Company, Ltd., 1962.

Chapter 3

The Roles of Grandparents:
The Use of Proverbs
in Value Transmission

Harriette P. McAdoo
Linda A. McWright

SUMMARY. This paper examines the roles of grandparents, the nature of relationships between them and their grandchildren, and the implications of the attachments inherent in such relationships. It further examines the methods of using proverbs by grandparents to transmit values to their grandchildren. Family oriented values and cultural values are passed down from generation to generation via oral tradition. This paper concludes with strong confirmation of developmental processes for grandchildren related to role functions performed between them and their grandparents.

Grandparents have important roles to play within their families that go beyond simply grandparenting alone. Their roles can be

---

Harriette Pipes McAdoo, PhD, is Professor with the Department of Family and Child Ecology at Michigan State University. Linda McWright is a PhD student with the Department of Family and Child Ecology, College of Human Ecology, Michigan State University.

Address correspondence to: Family and Child Ecology, Michigan State University, 101 Morrill Hall, East Lansing, MI 48824.

[Haworth co-indexing entry note]: "The Roles of Grandparents: The Use of Proverbs in Value Transmission." McAdoo, Harriette P., and Linda A. McWright. Co-published simultaneously in *Activities, Adaptation & Aging* (The Haworth Press, Inc.) Vol. 19, No. 2, 1994, pp. 27-38; and: *Aging Families and Use of Proverbs for Values Enrichment* (ed: Vera R. Jackson) The Haworth Press, Inc., 1994, pp. 27-38. Multiple copies of this article/chapter may be purchased from The Haworth Document Delivery Center [1-800-3-HAWORTH; 9:00 a.m. - 5:00 p.m. (EST)].

27

observed in the transmission of families values, beliefs, and cultural norms through the use of their wisdom that extends beyond their life span. One of the most important roles that grandparents play is to bridge the family history of the past, through their lifetime, into the memories of their grandchildren and into the future. The transmission of family values, to those within their family, is crucial to the maintenance of culture within the lives of families. The values that are espoused by family members may change over time, but the core of beliefs that underbridge families become the cultural foundation that makes families unique, yet they tie them into a system of ethnic, religious, and national mores that bring out the cultural dimensions of families.

The current paper focuses on the roles of grandparents, the nature of the relationship between grandparents and grandchildren, as well as the implications of the attachments in such a relationship. It looks at the transmission of the value of connectedness and the relationships of grandparents and grandchildren through the use of proverbs. Proverbs, "little" expressions, repeated sayings, and parables are the primary modes of cultural maintenance and transmission of family values.

While all family and cultural groups transmit values, the African American experience from Africa to North America, and from enslavement to the present, has relied heavily on the oral tradition and not upon the written word. African Americans have prevailed in the oral transmission of culture via the use of proverbs and "little" sayings that are repeated over and over to their grandchildren.

THE ROLES OF GRANDPARENTS

A key role that grandparents play is simply being present. The presence of grandparents serves as a comfort to both adult children and grandchildren (Hagestad, 1985). For grandchildren, grandparents often serve as a source of companionship, confidants, and advice-givers (Daliman-Jenkins Papalia, & Lopez, 1987). Their role is to maintain the family system (Troll, 1983). Cross-culturally, grandparents serve important stabilizing functions in the wider family system. They provide a wide range of support to their children and grandchildren in times of crisis (Cherlin & Furstenberg, 1986;

Johnson, 1988; Troll, 1983). In their parent role, they bolster their children through encouragement, as well as emotional and financial support (Bengston & Robertson, 1985).

Neugarten and Weinstein (1964) found that grandparents view themselves within the framework of five structural types:

1. Formal: Grandparents follow a prescribed role, maintain constant interest in the child, and maintain well-documented lines between parenting and grandparenting.
2. Fun-seeker: Informality, playfulness, and mutuality of satisfaction characterize the relationship.
3. Surrogate parent: A grandmother-identified role, in which she assumes caretaking responsibilities for children at the initiative of an adult daughter.
4. Reservoir of family wisdom: A grandfather-identified role as dispenser of special skills and resources; lines of authority between generations are clearly marked.
5. Distant figure: Contact with the child is infrequent, although the grandparent is benevolent.

These studies show the significance of the emotional attachments and connectedness between grandparents and grandchildren. The attachment is unique in that the relationship is exempt from the psycho-emotional intensity and responsibility that exists in parent/child relationships (Kornhaber & Woodward, 1981). The love, nurturance, and acceptance that grandchildren have found in the grandparent/grandchild relationship, confers a natural form of social immunity on children which they cannot get from any other person or institution (Kornhaber & Woodward, 1981). However, a grandparent or grandchild's perception of this relationship may differ or vary from the above findings, depending on the age or time of transition into grandparenthood.

During the past decade, there has been increasing recognition of the importance of grandparents as a stabilizing force in multigenerational families (Johnson, C. L., 1988). Recently, grandparents have become central to family dynamics, and they serve as a family resource and are the transmitters of family values. These values connect generation to generation (McAdoo, 1991), from grandparents to grandchildren. Much of value transmission takes place through proverbs. Grandparents skillfully pass on wisdom and survival skills without the child's conscious awareness (Troll, 1983; Barranti, 1985). Grandparents of today fulfill a number of roles within the family.

More people are living long enough to become grandparents. American grandparents are living longer, as a result of reductions in mortality rates and increased control over childhood diseases. The average age of becoming a grandparent in the United States is the mid to late forties. There are 31.8 million people 65 years or older in the United States. They represent 12.6% of the population. The number of older Americans increased by 6.1 million or 24% since 1980. In 1990, 81% of persons 65 and over were White, 8% were Black, 4% were Hispanic and 3% were other races. The older population is expected to continue to grow and by the year 2030 there will be about 66 million older adults, more than twice the 1990 number (AARP, 1992).

The majority (65%) of older adults live in a family setting and 4 out of 5 have living children. Sixty-six percent live within 30 minutes of a child. About 15% were living with their children, other relatives and nonrelatives. The increase in life expectations and living arrangements suggest older adults are living longer, are involved in family networks and interact with their children and grandchildren.

Due to a decrease in fertility, there are fewer grandchildren to go around. However, most grandparents live in close proximity to at least one of the children, and have regular contact with children and grandchildren. Cherlin and Furstenberg (1986) indicated that grandparents become parent-like figures when they live close by, and provide assistance and emotional or moral support. Modern grandparents can keep in touch with their grandchildren more easily than grandparents of previous ages, and they have more time to devote to them. Their grandchildren may, in turn, need them more.

While the time of entry into grandparenthood has not undergone dramatic change, its sequencing relative to other role changes shows new patterns. Reduction of the age at which women finish their childrearing has made it rare to find overlap between active parenting and grandparenting status. The two roles have become more clearly sequenced in the life course, than was the case when women bore children throughout their fertile years. Then middle-aged women were often still occupied with childrearing after their oldest children had already made them grandmothers.

Whether mothers are off-schedule or on-time in their transition to grandparenthood, grandparents cross-culturally, are now playing a crucial role in family transitions, such as underemployment and unemployment, divorce, and substance abuse by their adult children.

Surrogate parenting, when the grandparent becomes the primary caretaker or parent, is becoming more prevalent; 5% of the children in the United States lived with grandparents in 1990. Surrogate grandparenting is more common among African American families than White families (Atchley, 1994). In addition to drugs, the spread of AIDS and the high incarceration of parents, there continues to be a need for grandparents to assume the primary parenting role in the future.

Many mothers in America enter the labor force when their children are only infants, or at best, of preschool age; and nearly half of all American children will experience their parents' divorce, and will spend an average of five years in a single-parent home (Edelman, 1987). Women of color, however, have traditionally been in the labor force, regardless of work status.

GRANDPARENTS' RELATIONS TO GRANDCHILDREN

Grandparents as caregivers or surrogate parents have received considerable attention (Kornhaber & Woodward, 1981; Tinsley & Parke, 1984). Divorce distress has resulted in the building of strong grandparent/grandchild relationships (Wilson & Deshane, 1982). Grandparents have functioned not only as surrogate parents, but as mediators of tension and anxiety.

An important contribution to the connectedness in the grandparent/grandchild relationship is that grandparents are in a position to offer grandchildren a form of unconditional love which parents, because of many other responsibilities, are unable to offer (Kornhaber & Woodward, 1981). The experience of being loved simply for being alive contributes to one's developing self-esteem and positive sense of self. Consequently, individuals who are loved, grow up to be loving people who, in turn, make positive contributions to society (Peck, 1978).

Grandparenthood provides a cushion of support that helps to absorb family pressure, diffuse social stresses, and provide needed aid and assistance (Harris & Associates, 1975; Kan & Antonucci, 1980; Kornhaber & Woodward, 1981). Experiencing positive emotional attachments can result in a developing sense of self-effectiveness, and this enables risk-taking behavior and creative adventuring throughout life (Kalish & Knudston, 1976). These psycho-emotional effects of the relationship can definitely enhance the quality of life for both grandchildren and grandparents.

During periods of crisis, grandparents often become actively involved in extending aid to the family. For example, Johnson (1988b) found that about 60 percent of the divorced adult children in her sample were dependent upon the parents for help. Gladstone (1988) discovered that contact between grandchildren and grandmothers increased after an adult child's separation or divorce. In addition, grandmothers in his sample reported that they provided more support (e.g., baby sitting) after the separation or divorce.

An in-depth study of the significance of connectedness in the grandparent/grandchild relationships by Kornhaber and Woodward (1981) revealed emotional attachment to be a fundamental component of the relationship for children. Using qualitative data, the authors identified several modes of attachment that existed between grandchildren and grandparents: (a) the grandparent as the essence of family bonds; (b) the grandparent as a constant object in the life of the children, who knew their grandparents through personal experience and through stories; (c) grandparents as teachers of basic skills; (d) grandparents as negotiators between child and parent, helping one to understand the other; (e) same-sexed grandparents as role models for adulthood (f) grandparents as determinants of how the young feel about the old in society; and, (g) grandparents as "great parents," providing a secure and loving adult/child relationship that is next in emotional power only to the relationship with parents. It can be proposed that these connecting entities between grandparent and grandchildren represent ways in which the grandparent/grandchild relationship functions as a resource for the family and its members.

Kornhaber and Woodward (1981) studied the roles of grandparents from the grandchild's perspective. The sample involved 300 grandchildren, 5 to 18 years of age, and five specific roles from the grandchild's perspective were identified. They are: (a) Historian: Grandparents provide both a cultural and familial sense of history; (b) Mentor: Grandparents offer wisdom, teach children to work with the basics of life, and deepen sex role identity; (c) Role Model: Grandparents serve as role models for the children's future role as a grandparent, for aging, and for family relationships; (d) Wizard: Grandparents are "magical" to children, telling stories and stroking the child's imagination; and, (e) Nurturer/Great Parent: The most basic role that grandparents play is widening the support system for children.

The distinction between how grandfathers function versus how grandmothers function needs to be examined. Stern, Dietz, and Kalof, in a study, looked at value orientation, gender and environmental concerns and they found significant differences between genders in terms of how they related to their immediate environments. They basically postulated that women tended to see a world of inherent interconnections. Men, on the other hand, tended to see the same world clearly separated, i.e., events abstracted from their contexts. The suggestions of their findings are that even when both held the same values, men tend to be less attentive than women to links between the environment and things they value. For grandparents it would appear that gender socialization may lead grandmothers to focus more on children's health and well-being, and grandfathers on children's economic well-being.

In the absence of a grandparent/grandchild relationship, it has been suggested that children experience a deprivation of nurturance, support and emotional security (Kornhaber & Woodward, 1981). Mead (1978) proposed that when an individual does not have intergenerational family connectedness, there is a resulting lack of a cultural and historical sense of self. Similarly, Baranowski (1982) viewed the lack of grandparent/grandchild connectedness as a central problem in the adolescent's attempt to resolve the developmental crisis of ego identity. He concluded that part of resolving the crisis involved developing a sense of one's uniqueness as well as one's continuity; the historical and ancestral significance experienced in intergenerational family relationships can contribute to this resolution.

GRANDPARENTS AS A RESOURCE
FOR INTERGENERATIONAL CONNECTEDNESS

Grandparents function as a family resource through intergenerational connectedness. One result of connectedness is the psycho-emotional experience of attachment between grandparent and grandchildren (Kornhaber & Woodward, 1981). Grandparents serve as connections between the past and future, giving a sense of historical and cultural rootedness. Grandparents function as a family resource for bridging the past, present and future for younger generations, giving them a sense of security, aiding in their ego development, and offering them a vision of the future (Baranowski, 1982; Kornhaber & Woodward, 1981). Much of the bridging between past and present is done via usage of proverbs.

Clearly, researchers have shown a relationship between those values embraced and held sacrosanct in our social system and those values held by families. Many of the social ills faced by our society can be traced directly to family values that are promulgated by grandparents and passed on to grandchildren. An investigation of values held and values transmitted allows one to carefully examine how culture is intergenerationally transmitted. Implicit in the discussion are findings by Dietz and Stern (in press) that the notion that value orientations may not be mutually exclusive, and that individuals may hold multiple orientations; and that value orientations may vary across individuals, social-structural groups, and culture.

The use of proverbs by grandparents has often taken the form of little sayings and the repeating of traditional proverbs. Many of these proverbs are based on the biblical sayings and traditional wisdom that has been repeated for generations. The lives of present grandchildren are often outside of the protective communities of the grandparents. The use of these proverbs are a means of connecting the grandchildren to the shared wisdom of the lives of their elders.

Researchers have discussed proverbs as part of the African American oral tradition (Finnegan, 1981; McAdoo, 1991). They viewed them as allusive and metaphorical images of their family values.

Page and Washington's (1987) study of intra-familial, transgenerational transmission of values found that the most highly valued and ranked proverbs were those that related connectedness, family security, true friendship and continuity. Page and Washington found that African American women valued these proverbs: (a) "What goes around comes around"; (b) "Blood is thicker than water"; (c) "Cleanliness is next to godliness"; and (d) "If you don't think anything of yourself, no one will." These proverbs represent the values these parents wanted to pass on to their children.

McAdoo's (1991) study of transgeneration values and outcomes for children clearly found that parents stress values that were family-oriented, that promoted self-sufficiency, self-esteem and positive racial attitudes. McAdoo found that African American parents valued these proverbs: (a) "Don't count your chickens before they are hatched"; (b) "One cannot live by bread alone"; (c) "What goes around comes around"; (d) "It's a poor dog that does not wag it's own tail"; (e) "The blacker the berry, the sweeter the juice."

Grandparents are primary promulgators of values transmission. These values tend to be transmitted through the usage of proverbs and collections of values, beliefs, attitudes, and behaviors. The use of proverbs occurs in the daily interactions with the grandchildren; as they comb their hair, discipline them at mealtimes, and as they bed them down at night. Grandparents may not even be aware that they are using these pat sayings. They see themselves as responding as they should, as they were responded to when they were children. The selection of proverbs says a great deal about where they were raised, the social class they belonged to, the racial group of their ascendants, and the religious memberships of their families.

Proverbs communicate African American family values, morality identification, self-preservation, coping skills, ancestry linkage and culture, regardless of social class or education (McAdoo, 1991; 1989). McAdoo's study clearly supported the hypothesis that family-oriented values are passed down from generation to generation via the use of proverbs and the oral tradition. Values related to self-sufficiency, self-esteem, and positive racial attitudes are all inherent in proverbs used by grandparents.

Grandparents serve the obvious functions associated with their presence and all of its inherent ramifications and implications. They serve as a family resource and provide intergenerational connectedness. Caring and nurturing are two of the more salient processes associated with the grandparenting function. Actively involved grandparents are needed because of the changes that have occurred in the age distribution of the population of the United States, longer life expectancies, decreased fertility, increases in single parenthood, the decreased ability of many men to support their families financially, joblessness, inadequate child care facilities, and teenage motherhood.

In summary, the roles that grandparents' play in the development of their grandchildren seems as critical as any other function that they perform. Grandparents contribute positively to future generations. They will have an influence on what the world will eventually look like, and how well its people will adjust. It is apparent from the literature that in an era of family growth the development not characterized by the nuclear family, but extended and single parent families, grandparents fulfill a critical and necessary function. They represent a "missing link" in the developmental process for many of American's children. They provide the connectedness and assure continuity in this developmental process.

There do not appear to be research studies available on the very important contribution of grandparents, and the transmission of values. Much of the literature assigns only traditional roles to grandparents. At the same time, it appears that there are broad, expansive, and in-depth roles for grandparents to play in shaping the future of our society. There is an obvious need for more empirical and conceptual studies that address issues of connectedness between grandparents and grandchildren, with more in-depth analysis of the implications and ramifications of this concept. Grandparents have played important roles in the transmission of values to grandchildren. As families undergo changes, their roles will be even greater in the future.

REFERENCES

American Association of Retired Persons. 1992. *A profile of older Americans: 1992*. Washington, D.C.: American Association of Retired Persons.
Atchley, R.D. 1994. *Social forces and aging: An introduction to social gerontology*. Belmont, CA: Wadsworth.

Baranowski, M.D. 1982. Grandparent-adolescent relations: Beyond the nuclear family. *Adolescence, 17,* 575-584.

Barranti, C.R. 1985. The grandparent/grandchild relationship: Family resource in an era of voluntary bonds. *Family Relations, 34,* 343-352.

Bengtson, V.L. & Robertson, J.F. (Eds.). 1985. *Grandparenthood.* Newbury Park, CA: Sage.

Cherlin, A.J., & Furstenberg, F.F. 1986. *The new American grandparent: A place in the family, a life apart.* New York: Basic Books.

Daliman-Jenkins, M., Papalia, D., & Lopez, M. 1987. Teenagers' reported interaction with grandparents; Exploring the extent of alienation. *Lifestyles: A Journal of Changing Patterns, 3-4,* 35-46.

Edelman. M.W. 1987. *Families in peril: An agenda for social change.* Cambridge, MA: Harvard University Press.

Finnegan, R. 1981. Proverbs in Africa: Oral literature in Africa. In W. Meider & A. Dundes (Eds.), *The wisdom of many: Essays on the proverb.* New York: Garland, 10-42.

Gladstone, J.W. 1988. Perceived changes in grandmother-grandchild relations following a child's separation or divorce. *The Gerontologist, 28,* 66-72.

Hagestad, G.O. 1985. Continuity and connectedness. In V. L. Bengtson and J. F. Robertson (Eds.), *Grandparenthood,* 31-48. Newbury Park, CA: Sage.

Harris, L. & Associates. 1975. *The myths and realities of aging in America.* Washington, D.C.: National Council on Aging.

Johnson, C.L. 1988. Active and latent functions of grandparenting during the divorce process. *The Gerontologist, 28,* 185-191.

Johnson, C.L. 1988b. Postdivorce reorganization of relationships between divorcing children and their parents. *Journal of Marriage and the Family,* 50, 221-231.

Kahn, R.L., & Antonucci, T.C. 1980. Convoys over the life course: Attachment, roles, and social support. In P. Baltes and O. Brim (Eds.), *Lifespan Development and Behavior, 3,* 253-286.

Kalish, R. & Knudston, F. 1976. Attachment versus disengagement: A lifespan conceptualization. *Human Development, 19,* 171-182.

Kornhaber, A. & Woodward, K. 1981. *Grandparent/grandchildren: The vital connection.* Garden City: Doubleday.

McAdoo, H.P. 1989. Transgenerational patterns of upward mobility in African American families. In H. P. McAdoo (Ed.), *Black families,* 148-167. Newbury Park, CA: Sage.

McAdoo, H. 1991. Family values and outcomes for children. *Journal of Negro Education, 60,* 361-365.

Mead, M. 1978. *Culture and commitment: The new relationship between the generations in the 1970s.* New York: Columbia.

Neugarten, B. & Weinstein, K. 1964. The changing American grandparent. *Journal of Marriage and the Family, 26,* 199-204.

Page, M.H. & Washington, N.D. 1987. Family proverbs and value transmission of single Black mothers. *Journal of Social Psychology, 127, 49-58.*

Peck. S. 1978. *The road less traveled.* New York: Simon and Schuster.

Stern, P.C. & Dietz, T. (in press). The values of environmental concern. *Journal of Social Issues.*

Stern, P.C., Dietz, T., & Kalof, L. 1993. Value orientations, gender, and environmental concern. Reprint from *Environment and Behavior,* May, 322-548.

Tinsley, B.R. & Parke, R.D. 1984. Grandparents as support and socialization agents. In M. Lewis (Ed.), *Beyond the dyad.* New York: Plenum Press, 161-194.

Troll, L.E. 1983. Grandparents: The family watchdogs. In T. H. Brubaker (Ed.), *Family relationships in later life.* Newbury Park, CA: Sage, 63-74.

Wilson, K.B. & DeShane, M.R. 1982. The legal rights of grandparents: A preliminary discussion. *The Gerontologist, 22,* 67-71.

PART III

HEALTH
AND REHABILITATION

Chapter 4

Efficacy of a Day Treatment Program in Management of Diabetes for Aging African Americans

Leo E. Hendricks
Rosetta T. Hendricks

SUMMARY. The thesis of this paper holds those aging African Americans with diabetes mellitus, who exercise godly wisdom in complying with a diabetes mellitus care day treatment program regimen, will experience better physical performance, less disability and pain, greater autonomy and self-sufficiency, personal growth, and greater social and spiritual connectedness.

This paper posits day treatment of diabetes among aging African Americans deserves special consideration because older adults are a neglected group in terms of diabetes education (Funnell, 1994); and because recent diabetes literature draws attention to the need for more specific and culturally sensitive diabetes care (Martinez,

Leo E. Hendricks, MSW, MRP, PhD, is President and CEO of Leo Hendricks Consulting Associates.

Rosetta T. Hendricks, MSN, RN, C, FNP, CDE, is Coordinator of a nationally recognized Diabetes Patient Education and Treatment Program, for the Department of Veterans Affairs Medical Center, Washington, DC.

Address correspondence to: 3055 Harrison Street, N.W., Washington, DC 20015.

[Haworth co-indexing entry note]: "Efficacy of a Day Treatment Program in Management of Diabetes for Aging African Americans." Hendricks, Leo E., and Rosetta T. Hendricks. Co-published simultaneously in *Activities, Adaptation & Aging* (The Haworth Press, Inc.) Vol. 19, No. 2, 1994, pp. 41-51; and: *Aging Families and Use of Proverbs for Values Enrichment* (ed: Vera R. Jackson) The Haworth Press, Inc., 1994, pp. 41-51. Multiple copies of this article/chapter may be purchased from The Haworth Document Delivery Center [1-800-3-HAWORTH; 9:00 a.m. - 5:00 p.m. (EST)].

1993). In addition, diabetes treatment of elderly African Americans is warranted because more people with diabetes are surviving to old age (Gitman, 1971). More recently, Lun (1993) noted the geriatric population represents an increasingly large proportion of the total population in the United States. More than 23 million Americans are 65 years of age and older and they represent more than 12 percent of the current population. It is projected that by the year 2030, the elderly population will grow to 52 million, representing 17 percent to 20 percent of the total population.

DIABETES DEFINED

There are three different classes of diabetes: non-insulin dependent diabetes mellitus, insulin dependent diabetes mellitus, and gestational diabetes mellitus, all characterized by glucose intolerance. This is the inability to properly use glucose, a form of sugar, whether eaten or produced by the body after a meal. The most common kind of diabetes is non-insulin dependent diabetes mellitus (NIDDM) or type II diabetes. NIDDM develops most often in adults over 40, especially those who are obese. People with this type of diabetes manage the disease through diet, weight control, and exercise, often accompanied by oral diabetes medication or insulin. Insulin dependent diabetes mellitus (IDDM) or type I diabetes is much less common and usually develops in children and young adults. People with IDDM must have regular insulin injections. Gestational diabetes is a mild form of diabetes that affects women only during pregnancy. Women who have had this form of diabetes are more likely to develop NIDDM when they are older. People with diabetes often have unusual thirst, frequent urination, fatigue, or an ill feeling (U.S. Department of Health and Human Services, 1986).

What is more, it has been confirmed in the literature that prevalence of diabetes mellitus is age-related, increasing nearly ninefold from about 2 percent in persons aged 20 to 44 years to about 18 percent in persons between 65 and 74 (Lun, 1993). Simon and Frishman (1993), too, have noted that even in the aged, the incidence of diabetes, almost all of which is non-insulin dependent mellitus (NIDDM) is increasing. Type II or non-insulin dependent diabetes accounts for 90 percent of the cases seen in the elderly (Lun, 1993). More specifically, Hendricks and Haas (1991) have pointed out that diabetes is 50-60 percent higher in African Americans than in white populations.

Diabetes and its complications kill thousands of people each year, and a large share of them are African Americans. Diabetes is the third leading cause of death from disease in the African American population, exceeded by heart disease and cancer (Hendricks and Haas, 1991). In fact, diabetes statistics reveal a wide health gap between minorities and non-minorities, according to the report of the Secretary's Task Force on Black and Minority Health (U.S. Department of Health and Human Services, 1986). For example, the Task Force pointed out that diabetes is 33 percent more common among African Americans than whites, and the picture is even worse for African American women. African American women have 50 percent more diabetes than white women and face greater risk if they are obese.

Additionally, the complications of diabetes also are more frequent in African Americans. Heart disease, stroke, kidney failure, and blindness—all are more common among African Americans with diabetes than among whites with diabetes. However, the Task Force quoted statistics showing good management of diabetes could prevent these complications in a large number of cases. For example:

- Controlling high blood pressure in people with diabetes could reduce strokes by 75 percent, coronary heart disease by 25 to 50 percent, and peripheral vascular disease (circulatory problems) by 30 to 60 percent.
- By quitting smoking, people with diabetes could reduce strokes by 5 percent, coronary heart disease by 10 percent, and peripheral vascular disease by 30 percent.
- Early diagnosis and treatment for proliferative retinopathy, an eye problem caused by diabetes, could reduce severe visual loss by more than 50 percent.
- Good foot care could reduce amputations by more than 50 percent (U.S. Department of Health and Human Services, 1986).

Therefore, good control of glucose levels in older patients with diabetes is important, since age interacts with diabetes to accelerate the onset of diabetic complications, which in turn have a devastating impact on morbidity and the quality of life in older individuals (Lun, 1993).

CONCEPT OF A DIABETES DAY TREATMENT PROGRAM FOR AGING AFRICAN AMERICANS

Since elderly African Americans use traditional health care services less than their white counterparts, an alternative means to diabetes treatment is suggested (Heckler, 1985). From available data (Anderson and Jenkins, 1994) and clinical experience, the authors think an elderly diabetes day treatment program would be efficacious in preventing or delaying the development and progression of complications in aging African Americans diagnosed with type II diabetes. As used here, an elderly diabetes day treatment program refers to a facility established to provide:

- Blood glucose monitoring
- Weight monitoring
- Foot care
- Low impact aerobic exercise
- Blood pressure monitoring
- Medication administration
- Socialization through informal group discussion around problems patients may have in achieving and maintaining their blood glucose levels between 140-180mg/dL
- Health referrals during daytime hours
- Lunch

Borrowing from Hunter (1992), at night, the clients return to their own homes with family or caregiver. "Elderly" means persons who have reached at least their 65th birthday.

Recommended staffing, for the proposed diabetes day treatment program, at a minimum would include:

- An adult or family nurse practitioner certified as a diabetes educator

- Dietitian
- Direct care providers

Clients are referred into the program by their primary care provider. On admission, the nurse practitioner obtains a health history and does a physical assessment, including a functional and mental status exam. Information gathered is used to guide the nurse practitioner in affording the best opportunity for aging African Americans to control diabetes and it complications. The treatment program is designed to serve eight clients, for four hours one day a week, over a period of seven months.

The authors' approach to diabetes control, for aging African Americans, encompasses the strategy of secondary prevention, that is, to prevent acute complications and the appearance of chronic complications through appropriate patient and professional education, therapy, and medical follow-up. Diabetes literature confirms that a prevention-oriented approach to diabetes is more effective than a crisis-oriented approach (U.S. Department of Health and Human Services, 1986).

EVALUATION OF THE DIABETES
DAY TREATMENT PROGRAM

The wisdom of the prudent is to understand
his [or her] way . . .

–Proverbs 14:8, KJV

A truly epidemiologic approach to the need of bringing health care to aging African Americans with diabetes, via a day treatment program, must be based on knowledge of whether the day treatment program is efficacious in promoting glucose control and the prevention of diabetes complications. Using criteria set forth in the literature (U.S. Department of Health and Human Services, 1986; Glasgow and Osteen, 1992), the efficacy of the authors' proposed diabetes day treatment program can be measured by demonstrating during valid sequential audits that some, and preferably all, of the following occur:

- Cessation of smoking
- Decreased sick days
- Decreased days of hospitalization
- Decreased morbidity (e.g., diabetic acidosis, amputations)
- Decreased mortality (increased duration of life)
- Decreased costs of evaluation, education, therapy, and follow-up
- Improved cholesterol levels
- Improved self-sufficiency
- Significant decrease in plasma glucose level in those with IDDM
- Significant decrease in weight and plasma glucose level in those with NIDDM
- Improved quality of life (better physical performance, less disability and pain, greater autonomy and self-sufficiency, personal growth, and greater social and spiritual connectedness)

A merry heart doeth good like a medicine: but a broken spirit drieth the bones

−Proverbs 17:22, KJV

More specifically, to promote quality of life for aging African Americans, a diabetes day treatment program must meet the elderly's primary needs. Maslow's Hierarchy of Needs theory applies to aging African Americans and other age groups (Maslow, 1943). The five levels of need are physiological, security and safety, love, self-esteem, and self-actualization. Each of these needs is addressed in planning a quality diabetes day care program for aging African Americans (Hunter, 1992).

Pleasant words are as an honeycomb, sweet to the soul, and health to the bones

−Proverbs 16:24, KJV

PATIENT ADHERENCE TO THE DIABETES DAY TREATMENT PROGRAM

Take fast hold of instruction; let her not go: keep her; for she is thy life

−Proverbs 4:13, KJV

However, optimum effectiveness of the diabetes treatment regimen usually depends upon the older adult performing the diabetes self-care behavior prescribed (Polly, 1992). Additionally, as noted by Hinnen (1993), " . . . diabetes care is complicated. It is expensive. It requires that the person with the diabetes be knowledgeable, have good cognitive and motor skills, be able to problem solve, and be motivated to implement self-management of the disease. Diabetes is controlled better when support people are involved actively with the person with the diabetes. A weak link in any of these areas may reduce adherence to the regimen."

Although most correlations were weak, the literature illustrates compliance decreases as the patients perceived more barriers to following the prescribed regimen. Compliance increased when patients keenly perceived the benefits of following the prescribed regimen (Selely, 1993). Moreover, adherence was associated positively with the "occurrence of symptoms, with continuity of care, with having a personal source of care, and with certain factors in the social context, including social support and stability of primary groups" (Rosenstock, 1985).

FACTORS PROMOTING ADHERENCE TO DIABETES REGIMEN

Apply thine heart unto instruction, and thine ears to the words of knowledge

–Proverb 23:12, KJV

Consistent with the literature (Anderson et al., 1991; Hinnen, 1993, Seley, 1993), and through her clinical experience in working with aging African Americans with diabetes, the author has observed the following to be associated with adherence to the diabetes treatment regimen:

* Allow the patient to draw upon their past experiences in helping them to cope with their diabetes
* Involve the patient in setting their diabetes educational goals and outcomes
* Include family member or significant other in the teachings
* Let the patient know that you care about them as a person

- Use simple words and sentences that convey personal benefits to the patients for their following the prescribed diabetes treatment regimen—that is use clear communication to answer the "what's in it for me" question for the patient.
- Be accessible and readily available to respond to their questions, problems, or concerns
- Follow-up frequently

FACTORS CONTRIBUTING TO THE BARRIERS OF ADHERENCE TO DIABETES REGIMEN

Buy the truth, and sell it not; also wisdom, and instruction, and understanding

—Proverbs 23:23, KJV

Also, the author's clinical experience has revealed that some of the existing barriers to one adhering to a diabetes treatment regimen include the following:

- Cost of diabetes care and supplies
- Complexity of diabetes treatment regimen
- Lack of understanding of diabetes food exchange list
- Lack of involvement in deciding diabetes educational goals and outcomes
- Low literacy

In addition, Anderson et al. (1991) have pointed out that potential barriers to improved health care and health for African Americans with diabetes include racism, lack of knowledge, incorrect beliefs, lack of access to health care, differing cultural values and priorities, and poverty. However, they add, equitable and accessible diabetes care and culturally sensitive diabetes education can foster empowerment by enabling African Americans with diabetes to take care of their health through the recognition and promotion of individual strengths and personal goals.

This would suggest, then, that effective diabetes treatment of aging African Americans requires a sensitivity to and recognition of their unique cultural values and needs. Diabetes educators and health care providers need to consider specific ethnic beliefs, customs, food patterns, and health care practices, with the goal of incorporating these cultural factors into a practical and beneficial treatment regimen (Raymond and D'Eramo-Melkus, 1993).

COMPLIANCE

The way of a fool is right in his own eyes: but he [or she] that hearkeneth unto counsel is wise

–Proverbs 12:15, KJV

Nevertheless, aging African Americans must practice what they are taught. Immediate application, practice, repetition, and positive reinforcement will simplify learning. Also, linking the diabetes educational content to something the older patient is familiar with will enhance learning (Hinnen, 1993). Older adults can make changes in behavior if provided with information, strategies, skills, and support (Funnell, 1994).

The wise shall inherit glory: but shame shall be the promotions of fools

–Proverbs 3:35, KJV

Moreover, as noted by the American Diabetes Association (1993), "a continuing care plan is an essential feature in the management plan of every patient with diabetes. At each visit, the patient's progress in achieving treatment goals should be evaluated, and problems that have occurred should be reviewed. If goals are not being met, both the goals and the treatment plan need to be reassessed."

Although intensive diabetes management can delay and may even prevent the long-term complications of diabetes among aging African Americans, Anderson et al. (1991) maintained that "a lasting improvement in the health care and health of Black people must include a commitment to educate more Black health professionals. The mainstream medical and other schools for preparing health-care professionals in the U.S. should make and maintain a commitment to the training of more Black . . . health-care professionals. Because emphasis in health care in the U.S. continues to shift toward health promotion, disease prevention, and the treatment of chronic disease, the ability of health-care professionals and patients to communicate and understand each other will become increasingly important."

He [or she] that handleth a matter wisely shall find good . . .
                                                    –Proverbs 16:20

AUTHOR NOTE

An epidemiologist, Dr. Leo E. Hendricks serves as a subject matter expert in research and epidemiology to 8(a) and small business consulting firms. He has published extensively in the fields of Black adolescent fathers, help-seeking behavior, and mental health, and is a recognized consultant in these areas.

Rosetta T. Hendricks has focused on the area of diabetes patient education and treatment for over nine years. She serves as the principal investigator for an ongoing research project entitled, "Non-Invasive Glucose Monitoring: Use of Near Infrared Light." As a certified diabetes educator, she has served as a consultant to the National Certification Board for Diabetes Educators.

REFERENCES

American Diabetes Association. (1993). Standards of medical care for patients with diabetes mellitus. *Diabetes Care,* 16, Supplement 2, 10-13.

Anderson, R.M., Herman, W.H., Davis, J.M., Freedman, R.P., Funnell, M.M., & Neighbors, H.W. (1991). Barriers to improving diabetes care for blacks. *Diabetes Care,* 14, 605-609.

Anderson, L.A. & Jenkins, C.M. (1994). Conclusions. *Diabetes Spectrum,* 7, 121-124.

Bible, King James Version.

Funnell, M.M. (1994). Commentary. *Diabetes Spectrum,* 7, 118-120.

Gitman, L.E. (1971). Diabetes mellitus in the aged. In *U.S. Department of Health, Education, and Welfare–Working with Older People: A Guide to Practice,* 4, 219-224.

Glasgow, R.E. & Osteen, V.L. (1992). Evaluating diabetes education: Are we measuring the most important outcomes? *Diabetes Care,* 15, 1423-1432.

Heckler, M.M. (1985). Report of the secretary's task force on black and minority health. *Executive Summary,* 1, 1-239.

Hendricks, R.T. & Haas, L.B. (1991). Diabetes in minority populations. *Nurse Practitioner Forum*, 2, 199-202.

Hinnen, D. (1993). Issues in diabetes education. *Nursing Clinics of North America*, 28, 113-119.

Hunter, S. (1992). Adult day care: promoting quality of life for the elderly. *Journal of Gerontological Nursing*, 18, 17-20.

Lun, W.S. (1993). Use of oral hypoglycemic agents in the elderly: Pharmacotherapeutic considerations. *Practical Diabetology*, 12, 10-13.

Martinez, N.C. (1993). Introduction. *Diabetes Spectrum*, 6, 94.

Maslow, A.H. (1943). A theory of human motivation. *Psychological Review*, 50, 370-396.

Polly, R.K. (1992). Diabetes health beliefs, self-care behaviors, and glycemic control among older adults with non-insulin dependent diabetes mellitus. *The Diabetes Educator*, 18, 321-327.

Raymond, N.R. & D'Eramo-Melkus, G. (1993). Non-insulin-dependent diabetes and obesity in the black and hispanic population: culturally sensitive management. *The Diabetes Educator*, 19, 313-317.

Rosenstock, I. M. (1985). Understanding and enhancing patient compliance with diabetes regimens. *Diabetes Care*, 8, 610-616.

Seley, J.J. (1993). Is noncompliance a dirty word? *The Diabetes Educator*, 19, 386-391.

Simon, N.R. & Frishman, W.H. (1993). Diabetes mellitus in the elderly: A modifiable risk factor for cardiovascular disease? *Practical Diabetology*, 12, 4-13.

U.S. Department of Health and Human Services. (1986). Chemical dependency and diabetes. *Report of the Secretary's Task Force on: Black and Minority Health*, 7, 189-374.

Chapter 5

An Autologous Blood Donor Base: The African-American Elderly

Mildred K. Fuller

SUMMARY. The role that the elderly (persons over 65 years of age) play in maintaining a safe and adequate blood supply through preoperative autologous blood denotation is chronicled. Tenets that have historically prohibited the use of homologous donor blood for persons in need of transfusion therapy is examined from the African-American perspective. Attempts are made to dispel certain myths that African-Americans have about transfusion practices. Predicated on the proverbial directive–*In all labor there is profit, But mere talk leads only to poverty* (Proverbs 14:23)–recruitment strategies are recommended that encourage the African-American elderly to participate in autologous blood programs.

An homologous donor is one who is donating blood that may be used by someone other than the donor. Conversely, a preoperative autologous blood donor is one who donates his/her blood during the month preceding an elective surgical operation. Should this person require a transfusion of blood or blood products during surgery, the autologous blood would then be reinfused. An advantage associated

Mildred K. Fuller, PhD, MT (ASCP), CLS (NCA), is Chairperson, Department of Community Health and Rehabilitation, School of Health Related Professions and Natural Sciences, Norfolk State University, Norfolk, VA 23504.

[Haworth co-indexing entry note]: "An Autologous Blood Donor Base: The African-American Elderly." Fuller, Mildred K. Co-published simultaneously in *Activities, Adaptation & Aging* (The Haworth Press, Inc.) Vol. 19, No. 2, 1994, pp. 53-60; and: *Aging Families and Use of Proverbs for Values Enrichment* (ed: Vera R. Jackson) The Haworth Press, Inc., 1994, pp. 53-60. Multiple copies of this article/chapter may be purchased from The Haworth Document Delivery Center [1-800-3-HA-WORTH; 9:00 a.m. - 5:00 p.m. (EST)].

with this procedure is that it eliminates many of the adverse effects associated with homologous blood transfusions, particularly the risks of immune reaction, hepatitis, and acquired immune deficiency syndrome (AIDS) transmission (Turgeon, 1989).

The perception of the lay community, and the African-American community in particular, that AIDS and blood donation are connected have caused a reluctance among donors to give blood. For as the teaching directs–*Do not withhold good from those to whom it is due, When it is in your power to do it* (Proverbs 3:27)–educational efforts are needed to overcome these obstacles in maintaining a safe and adequate blood supply. Moreover, efforts should be directed toward recruiting a new group of donors that was previously considered as unsuitable donors–the elderly African-American.

AUTOLOGOUS BLOOD DONATION

The literature indicates that few studies have focused on the healthy, middle-class, well-educated, and health conscious elderly as blood donors, in general. This gap of information may help to explain the underrecruitment of the healthy elderly as either homologous or autologous blood donors. Elderly may be descriptive of one who is "rather old" and possesses "characteristics of later life" (*Webster's Dictionary*). Cassel and Brody (1990) have reported, based on current demographic trends, that between the years 1985 to 2000, the proportion of individuals over age 65 will have risen from approximately 11 percent to at least 17 percent of the overall population. As the elderly use at least 25 percent of the nation's blood supply, these data further suggest that the increase of the elderly in the population will be accompanied by an increased demand for blood transfusions (Pindyck, Avorn, Kuriyan, Reed, Iqbal, & Levine, 1987).

The current blood donation screening procedure, designed to protect the health of the potential donor as well as that of the recipient, appears to work equally well for the elderly population and younger persons. Simon, Rhyne, Wayne, and Garry (1991) screened 325 potential elderly blood donors, whose ages ranged from 63 to 77, by using the United Blood Services standard screening questionnaire. Of the screened population, 272 (83.7%) were eligible blood donors. Notably, this standard questionnaire disqualified the elderly from donating blood for the same reasons that it disqualified any other donor.

Yomtovian, Ceynar, Kepner, and Buhl (1987) provide comparative data on donor deferral rates. In this study, 224 donor-patients participated in an autologous donor program. Forty-one percent of the donors were over the age of 65, but only 5.8 percent were deferred for medical reasons. The average deferral rate for homologous blood donors has been reported as 11.9 percent (Tomasulo, 1980). These results lend support to the notion that the elderly is an underutilized volunteer donor base, and that the current donor screening protocol is efficient.

A major concern of the elderly participation as blood donors is death during phlebotomy. Mortality data for 1976 to 1985 indicate that there were only three donor deaths for over one million blood donations. These three donors were all under the age of 50 (Sazama, 1990). Another recognition, concerning the elderly, is that older blood donors have had more chances of being exposed to agents of disease. However, there is no evidence for the transmission of agents that cause cancer, heart disease or arthritis that is commonly seen in the elderly. Further, blood in the elderly is not "old" blood. Red blood cells, which gives the circulating blood its color, are removed from the bloodstream and replaced with new ones every few days in all normal human beings (Schmidt, 1991).

Unlike homologous blood donation, autologous blood donation depends primarily on the recruitment of physicians rather than patients. Surgeons or referring cardiologists are often recruited by transfusion therapy centers to encourage their patients to enroll in autologous donor programs. Patient-donors must meet the surgical procedure prerequisites of (1) a time span of approximately one month preoperatively during which the patient may donate; and (2) one in which red blood cell transfusion is expected. Typical surgical operations that would be considered for autologous donations include: hip replacement, coronary artery by-pass, aortofemoral by-pass, and hysterectomy for chronic pelvic inflammatory disease or endometriosis (Kruskall, Glazer, Leonard, Wilson, Pacini, Donovan, & Ransil, 1986; Toy, 1988).

Toy (1988) lists patient-selection criteria for autologous donation to include: a hemoglobin 11 g/dl or greater; hematocrit 34% or greater; capacity to generate red blood cells (adequate erythropoiesis); capacity to tolerate an acute 10-15% reduction in total blood volume; capacity to tolerate a possible vasovagal reaction; and no age limitation (Turgeon, 1989, p. 38). Autologous donors are advised that the interval between donations is usually one week with the final unit to be drawn within 72 hours of the anticipated operation or transfusion. Also, donations should be no more frequent than once every four days; and that predeposit phlebotomy should not be performed within 72 hours of major surgery. With daily oral iron supplements, the donor may donate up to eight units of whole blood within 20 days without ill effects (Bryant, 1994).

Autologous blood may be used to provide blood products to patients who refuse blood from homologous donors because of religious tenets. In these cases, the blood bank physician consults with the donor-patient's physician to determine the patient's eligibility for the autologous donation program. With the donor-patient's signed, informed consent, autologous blood recovery may be undertaken. This procedure requires the setting up of a "continuous loop" whereby the patient is connected to the recovery unit, which in turn is connected via an intravenous line back to the patient (Champion & Champion, 1993). Indeed, as the scripture suggests—

Prepare plans by consultation, and make war by wise guidance
—Proverbs 20:18

religious tenets, that have been barriers to the use of homologous donor blood for patients in need of transfusion therapy, will be eradicated with autologous blood use.

Autologous donation has gained in popularity since preoperative patients and their physicians have become more concerned about the risk of transmission of blood-borne infectious diseases in homologous blood. This trend has not been documented in the literature for African-Americans. Thus, efforts directed toward recruiting a new group of donors that was previously considered as unsuitable as donors—the elderly African-American—should be targeted. This donor cohort is at low risk for AIDS, have high iron stores, and tend to have more time available for blood donation.

RECRUITMENT STRATEGIES

Blood donation is both a civic and humanitarian obligation of all healthy individuals. It is, also, an altruistic action that should be encouraged by health providers on a regular basis (Mosley, 1991). Mayo (1992) suggested that the adequacy and safety of the blood supply are two integrally related issues. Recruitment strategies that encourage too many individuals to donate could result in an increased number of donors at risk for transfusion-transmissible disease. Thus, an adequate blood supply would be maintained but it may be unsafe. In contrast, if recruitment strategies did not motivate enough individuals to donate, the blood supply may be safe but inadequate (Mayo, 1992).

Giving heed to the adage

> Give instruction to a wise man, and he will be still wiser,
> Teach a righteous man, and he will increase his learning
> —Proverbs 9:9

clinicians have studied ways to increase the number of volunteer blood donors from a normative perspective. Schwartz and Tessler (1972) found that one's attitude contributed significantly to the prediction of intentions. Further, Pomazal and Jaccard (1976) found a strong relationship between expressed intentions and actual blood donation. These researchers queried potential blood donors about their intention to donate blood. Of the individuals expressing an intention to donate, 34% became blood donors. Conversely, of those who intended not to donate, only 1.9% actually became blood donors. Clearly, these data suggest that theoretical approaches are necessary for understanding the process of commitment to blood donation. Theoretical frameworks that have been widely applied to donor motivation and recruitment are the social cognitive theory (Bandura, 1986), reasoned action theory (Fishbein & Ajzen, 1975), attribution theory (Kelley, 1967) and role-identity theory (McCall & Simmons, 1978). Collectively, these theories provide knowledge on the processes by which both personal and situational factors impact the motivation, and behavior of blood donors (Piliavin, 1990).

Modeling is a process whereby one learns by observing the

action of others (Piliavin, 1990, p. 451). The literature suggests that "modeling" is an approach that affects blood donation decisions. Rushston and Campbell (1978) demonstrated through an experimental study the impact of modeling on blood donation decisions. In this study, each young female was paired with an older female. When the twosome were recruited to be blood donors, the likelihood of both persons actually donating blood increased when the older female was asked first to be a blood donor.

RECOMMENDATIONS

Research is needed to translate the insights gained from the theories on blood donor motivation and behavior into usable approaches for recruiting and retaining African-American blood donors. The following strategies are proposed:

1. Conduct an experimental study to determine the impact of incentive use on African-American blood donor retention.
2. Provide educational information that dispel fears and other excuses for non-donation, and study the impact of this strategy on African-American participation in blood programs.
3. Reduce the inconvenience of the blood donor process by making bloodmobiles more accessible to the targeted group.
4. Encourage modeling by making presentations to small groups of African-Americans about the importance of blood and its components. These steps would be taken to increase the group's awareness of community need, and to motivate them to become regular blood donors. This approach would be applicable to all healthy potential blood donors.
5. Target the healthy, elderly African-American with blood donor literature. As an outreach project, medical technology students and faculty from predominately black colleges and universities could provide this service to churches, and various civic groups with large numbers of African-Americans.

CONCLUSION

The maintenance of an adequate and safe blood supply is a shared responsibility. For as the biblical teaching admonishes–You may say that it is none of your business, but God knows and judges your motives.

He keeps watch on you; He knows. And He will reward you according to what you do

—Proverbs 24:12

It behooves each of us to acknowledge our sense of community and to work cooperatively in the recruitment of healthy blood donors.

REFERENCES

Bandura, A. (1986). *Social foundations of thought and action: A social cognitive theory.* Englewood Cliffs, NJ: Prentice-Hall.

Bible, King James Version.

Bryant, N. J. (1994). *An introduction to immunohematology.* Philadelphia, PA: W. B. Saunders Company.

Cassel, C. K. & Brody, J. A. (1990). Demography, epidemiology, and aging. In *Geriatric medicine* (pp. 16-27). Cassel, C. K., Riesenberg, D. E., Sorensen, L. B., & Walsh, J. R. (Eds.). New York: Springer-Verlag.

Champion, M. E. & Champion, M. S. (1993). Autologous blood recovery a guide for health care providers. *Physician Assistant, 17*(9), 55-59.

Fishbein, M. & Ajzen, I. (1975). *Belief, attitude, intention and behavior: An introduction to theory and research.* Reading, MA: Addison-Wesley.

Kelley, H. H. (1967). Attribution theory in social psychology. In Levine, D. (ed.) *Nebraska symposium on motivation* (Vol. 14, pp. 192-241). Lincoln, NE: University of Nebraska.

Kruskall, M. S., Glazer, E. E., Leonard, S. S., Willson, S. C., Pacini, D. G., Donovan, L. M. & Ransil, B. J. (1986). Utilization and effectiveness of a hospital autologous preoperative blood donor program. *Transfusion, 26*(4), 335-340.

Mayo, D. J. (1992). Evaluating donor recruitment strategies (editorial). *Transfusion, 32*(9), 797-799.

McCall, G. J. & Simmons, J. L. (1978). *Identities and interactions.* New York: The Free Press.

Mosley, J. W. (1991). Who should be our blood donor? (editorial). *Transfusion, 31*(8), 684-685.

Piliavin, J. A. (1990). Why do they give the gift of life? A review of research on blood donors since 1977. *Transfusion, 30*(5), 444-459.

Pindyck, J., Avorn, J., Kuriyan, M., Reed, M., Iqbal, M. J., & Levine, S. J. (1987). Blood donation by the elderly. Clinical and policy considerations. *Journal of the American Medical Association, 257,* 1186-1188.

Pomazal, R. & Jaccard, J. (1976). An informational approach to altruistic behavior. *Journal of Personality and Social Psychology, 33*, 317-326.

Rushton, J. P. & Campbell, A. C. (1978). Modeling, vicarious reinforcement and extraversion and blood donating in adults: Immediate and long term effects. *European Journal of Social Psychology, 7*, 251-268.

Sazama, K. (1990). Reports of 355 transfusion associated deaths: 1976 through 1985. *Transfusion, 30*, 583-590.

Schmidt, P. J. (1991). Blood donation by the healthy elderly (editorial). *Transfusion, 31*(8), 681-683.

Schwartz, S. H. & Tessler, R. C. (1972). A test of a model for reducing measured attitude-behavior discrepancies. *Journal of Personality and Social Psychology, 24*, 225-236.

Simon, T. L., Rhyne, R. L., Wayne, S. J., & Garry, P. J. (1991). Characteristics of elderly blood donors. *Transfusion, 31*(8), 693-697.

Tomasulo, P. A. et al. (1980). A study of criteria for donor deferral. *Transfusion, 20*, 511-518.

Toy, P. (1988). Preoperative autologous blood donation. *The American Association of Blood Banks Master Speaker Series–3 and 4.*

Turgeon, M. L. (1989). *Fundamentals of immunohematology*. Philadelphia: Lea & Febiger.

Yomtovian, R., Ceynar, J., Kepner, J. L., & Buhl, M. (1987). Predeposit autologous blood transfusion: An analysis of donor attitudes and attributes. *Quarterly Research Bulletin*, 45-50.

Chapter 6

From an African American Perspective–
Living with Disabilities After Age 50:
Learning Anew and Moving Forward

Roger D. Ford
Janice E. Smith

SUMMARY. For as long as we can remember, we've heard the saying that "you can't teach an old dog new tricks," interpreted to mean that it's difficult for people to break old habits and learn new things that will improve their lives. The authors look at this "proverb" or adage and prove that this is not always the case when it comes to the disabled elderly who are determined to remain productive and live life to its fullest with their families and in their communities. The authors show that for those who transcend the four barriers of apathy, mobility issues, lack of information and resistance to the new, especially assistive technology, life offers many opportunities and rewards. These barriers are examined from an African American perspective, as disability issues are affected by the variables of race and age.

Roger D. Ford has served as Executive Director of the District of Columbia Center for Independent Living for three years.

Janice E. Smith is a freelance writer and communications consultant, with more than 15 years of professional experience.

Address correspondence to: The D.C. Center for Independent Living, 1400 Florida Avenue, N.E., Suite 3, Washington, DC 20002.

[Haworth co-indexing entry note]: "From an African American Perspective–Living with Disabilities After Age 50: Learning Anew and Moving Forward." Ford, Roger D., and Janice E. Smith. Co-published simultaneously in *Activities, Adaptation & Aging* (The Haworth Press, Inc.) Vol. 19, No. 2, 1994, pp. 61-71; and: *Aging Families and Use of Proverbs for Values Enrichment* (ed: Vera R. Jackson) The Haworth Press, Inc., 1994, pp. 61-71. Multiple copies of this article/chapter may be purchased from The Haworth Document Delivery Center [1-800-3-HAWORTH; 9:00 a.m. - 5:00 p.m. (EST)].

YOU CAN'T TEACH AN OLD DOG NEW TRICKS, EH? OH, BUT YOU CAN

Sixty-two year-old Clara B. is not sure that there was any one thing that led her to put her anger aside after two years of passive resistance, and venture into her kitchen that day. But she's kept moving forward ever since. Ms. B. (Interview, 1994) today, is a vibrant woman, who gets around with a walker. With a ready smile and quick wit, she has once again taken charge of her own life.

However, she freely admits that for two years after a debilitating stroke, she was depressed and angry, so "I would just sit where they put me. I wanted to know why this happened to me. I'd always taken care of myself, done things the right way—never depended on either of my husbands."

The anger, which Ms. B. talked about, is typical of many of the disabled African American senior citizens that the District of Columbia Center for Independent Living (DCCIL) serves. But what is really more significant is that Ms. B. and others like her are living testaments who shatter the engraved in stone adage: "You can't teach an old dog new tricks."

At the DCCIL, they make it their business to "teach old dogs new tricks." But in order to do that, DCCIL has found that there are four major barriers that the elderly disabled must overcome. In addition to anger often exhibited in the form of apathy, the three other major obstacles are: lack of information about available resources; mobility/transportation and resistance to starting over, especially with assistive technology.

Founded in April 1981, DCCIL is a nonprofit, nonresidential, consumer and community based organization that assists persons with disabilities to realize their full potential. Primary funding comes from Title VII of the Rehabilitation Services Act of 1973 as amended, through the U.S. Department of Education, with matching funds provided by the Government of the District of Columbia's Department of Human Services, Rehabilitation Services Administration. Approximately 40 percent of the consumers serviced by DCCIL are senior citizens, 55 and over, and the majority are minorities, primarily African Americans.

To go further into this discussion, it is necessary to first define disability. A generally accepted definition of disability (Wilson, 1988) is that it is "any limitation experienced by a person who has any deviation from the normal, which results in defective function, structure, organization or development of the whole, or of any faculties, senses, systems or organs as compared with the activities of unimpaired individuals of similar age, sex, sub-culture and culture."

While we know that all four of the factors which inhibit disabled African Americans from successfully participating in rehabilitation are prevalent among the disabled of all ages and ethnic groups, these problems appear to be more pronounced among the African American elderly because of certain socio-economic elements. Various reports have shown that a smaller percentage of Blacks graduate from high school and colleges than whites and Blacks' earning power is below that of whites. Also, African Americans with disabilities often feel that becoming disabled is just another undeserved strike against them, making their apathy a chasm to bridge and exacerbating their resistance to use technological devices that could make their adjustment more comfortable.

Nationwide, the average African American adult with a disability is 42 years old, has less than a high school level of education, does not work, nor is actively seeking employment. In 1980, income from all sources was under $3,000. (Bowe, 1985).

Overall, African Americans with disabilities are less successfully rehabilitated in vocational programs. In comparing Black and white participation in rehabilitation, Atkins and Wright reported that compared to whites, Black vocational rehabilitation applicants were not only more likely to be screened out (found ineligible) but if made eligible for service, Blacks were less likely to be rehabilitated (Atkins, 1988). Consequently to adequately service African Americans, one cannot ignore race and social factors.

"Overall, public policies and programs of service delivery for Americans with disabilities have been designed for the general population and have not adequately benefitted people with disabilities from minority populations. Even the passage of the ADA may not, by itself, have a substantial impact on minorities unless both the minority and majority communities become much more aware of, and sensitive to, the needs of minorities with disabilities" (Wright and Leung, 1993).

Traditional counseling has its roots in traditional theories of counseling focusing on middle class persons. Yet, data show that many African Americans with disabilities are living in poverty (Atkins, 1988).

Now to the second variable of age: There is very little research on the element of age and disability. What is known is that "Taking age of onset into account is important for understanding the particular life circumstances, tasks and problems with which the individual with a disability must cope; however, age of onset as such does not appear to be a decisive factor governing the psychological outcome of the adjustment process" (Wright, 1983).

Moving to the first barrier to "learning new tricks," the lack of information about available resources–for rehabilitation, financial assistance, emotional support: "Black Americans with disabilities need information that is empowering. They need to know that they have rights as Americans that are not diminished because they are black or because they have disabilities, and especially not because they are both black and disabled. It is not sufficient to tell our clients about services that they may be entitled to receive. It is crucial to ensure that individuals know about their specific rights as clients of the social service systems they use and the resources available to ensure that those rights are upheld. It is only then that they can make informed choices and begin to take control of their lives" (Galiber, 1988).

In looking at aging and disability, it is necessary to be aware of two different groups: (1) those who are disabled after becoming elderly and (2) those who are already disabled before becoming senior citizens.

Oftentimes, disabled African Americans do not have access to information and resources that help their adjustment to living with a disability. Take the case of Barbara P. (Interview, 1994), who will fall into the latter group of an individual who is already disabled and will have to cope with advancing age.

Ms. P., 47, has multiple sclerosis, and is the caretaker for three grandchildren. A high school dropout, she worked in low paying jobs, sometimes two at a time, to take care of her own three children. When she first started having trouble with her feet and legs, she contends that her complaints were casually addressed by doctors and the health care system because she did not have private health insurance.

She tells of going to one health care provider about a foot ailment and being told to go back to work. She left, and headed to work, wrapping her leg in a plastic bag to keep it dry from the snow.

Ms. P. recounts a long story of numerous visits to various doctors before her illness was even diagnosed. Although MS is viewed as difficult to diagnose in general, rightly or wrongly, Ms. P. feels that she was given short shrift because she was a poor, black woman on Medicaid.

When she looks toward old age: She says if she's still living, "I see me suffering." What pushes her on, she says is the recognition that her grandchildren–ages 1, 4, and 9–are depending on her for the love, shelter and care their drug-addicted mother–Ms. P.'s daughter–is unable to provide.

Ms. P., who must use a wheelchair for mobility, has accepted the challenge, with some angst. While DCCIL is searching for wheelchair accessible housing for her, she lives in an apartment building that limits her mobility. In the past, she admits to giving away some of her food stamps to persons to get them to physically help her get in and out of her apartment.

Ms. P. is emphatic that the disabled need more information about available resources in order to help them make responsible decisions about their rehabilitation.

Indeed, mobility/transportation is the second big issue for the elderly with disabilities. In terms of mobility/transportation, two things must be examined–the individual's own fear of falling and failing, and especially for the elderly, a perceived fear of crime and harm in the world outside.

In discussing crime at the Washington, D.C. Mayor's Conference on Aging two years ago, it was noted (Green, 1992) that "The many needs, desires and fears of senior citizens in the District of Columbia do not differ from the needs, desires and fears of the elderly citizens in any other major city in the United States. They need to feel safe from violence and abuse in their own homes. They desire protection from crime while at home or walking the streets to their local supermarket. They fear that someone will take from them something very precious–their money, property, health, self-esteem–even their lives."

Green (1992) also pointed out that among the issues identified as critical to the well-being of the senior population in the District of Columbia were fear of assault while at home (homebound elderly) and fear of robbery or assault while traveling about the neighborhood (Green, 1992).

To address the issue of mobility, DCCIL provides door-to-door transportation for its consumers who cannot utilize public transportation–to medical and social service appointments, recreational activities and other events. While no fee is charged, donations are accepted, but service is limited because DCCIL has only two vans.

With the local public transit system coming into compliance with the American with Disabilities Act's transportation requirements, paratransit travel is available for the disabled. However helpful this might be, it still does not provide assistance for the disabled person from his or her home to the sidewalk, to combat the real or perceived fear of crime and falling out of ear's reach of someone to help.

As great a role as lack of information and mobility/transportation issues play in helping the elderly to adapt and move on with their lives, the last two factors–apathy and resistance–play even greater roles.

The suddenness of the onset of the disease and productivity of its course affect the older person's ability to adapt and incorporate changes into his or her everyday life (Strauss et al. 1984; Cott and Wilkins, 1993). In other words, the senior citizen's acceptance of change in dealing with a disability may have more to do with how the disability occurs than his or her age at the time.

For example, chronic illness and disability are seen as normative by elderly people themselves (Charmag, 1991; Belgrave, 1990). Consequently, the elderly may not seek attention for health problems but instead accept disability due to chronic illness as an inevitable part of growing older. Sluggish with apathy, which in part may be generated by anger, they refuse to seek help in making efforts to live with their disabilities. In some cases, these views of the inevitability of disability for the aged are shared by health care providers and families who permit the elderly person with disabilities to languish (Cott and Wilkins, 1993).

To look at this premise, we'll review the stories of Clara B., who suffered a sudden onset of disability following a stroke, and Oscar P., whose disability came about as a result of chronic illness and had the opportunity to adjust to its prognosis (Interviews, 1994).

It was a late Friday afternoon, on July 1, and Ms. B. was packing up her desk for the weekend, at the Federal Bureau of Prisons where she worked. She heard the phone ringing, but for some reason she couldn't lift her hand to pick it up. Then she realized she couldn't move her leg.

Her paralyzing stroke kept her in three hospitals for over three months. "In fact, they didn't think I would ever walk again. I had no strength on my left side—that kind of deflated me."

By her own account, Ms. B. said she became so distraught she thought about committing suicide. "I was just going to starve myself to death—I wasn't going to eat."

"I wanted to know why this had happened to me. I had always been so independent. I couldn't stand the idea of someone bathing me."

Her anger manifested itself in apathy. Day after day, hour after hour, she would sit at home, where she was placed by caring family members. Her younger son even moved in to stay with her. "I was in a lot of depression—I was just there." After two years of feeling sorry for herself, Ms. B. decided to rid herself of the anger, and reached down within to draw on the strengths that had taken her through much of her life.

On the other hand, Oscar P., now 56, had been challenged by diabetes for years. His doctor had told him of the possibility that his leg might have to be amputated. Thus, he says that he did not feel the apathy and anger, often experienced by persons who experience the onset of a sudden disability.

"I couldn't say I was ready for it, but it was something that had to be done." Because he had an early prognosis, Mr. P. says, "I had already made up my mind that it wasn't going to stop me."

Mr. P. acknowledges that because he didn't like the idea of himself with a cane or walker, he quickly learned to adapt to using his prosthetics (in this case an artificial limb). "Now I walk four miles a day."

Unfortunately, not all of the elderly are as receptive to assistive technology as Mr. P. Simply put, assistive technology is "tools used by individuals with disabilities such as wheelchairs, hearing aids, canes, crutches, walkers or other tools to enhance daily living"(DCPAT, 1993).

The DCCIL has found that elderly consumers often protest mightily against using assistive technology–sometimes out of anger that at this stage in their lives they have to learn how to do old things a new way–sometimes from fear of failing or feeling embarrassed in front of family and friends.

The D.C. Partnership for Assistive Technology (1993) says there are a number of misconceptions that may encourage resistance to seeking the help of assistance technology.

Myth: Assistive technology is the "be all and end all."

Fact: Assistive technology is a powerful tool useful to persons with disabilities in many ways and situations. But technology alone doesn't end all the difficulties that come with having a disability. Yet, assistive technology devices can make accomplishing a task easier.

Myth: Assistive Technology is complicated (high tech) and expensive.

Fact: Although some of the technology used today is complicated and expensive, some of the best solutions to assistive technology needs are simple, inexpensive and low tech.

Myth: A user's assistive technology requirements only need to be assessed once.

Fact: A particular device may be useful to a person with a disability for the rest of their life or for only a few months or years. As individuals expand their activities to encompass home, school, work and community, they may have new or different needs in these settings.

Myth: Assistive technology is just a luxury.

Fact: For someone with a disability who relies upon assistive technology to perform a critical function to achieve a desired goal in life, assistive technology is very much a necessity.

Myth: Only persons with certain types of disabilities find assistive technology useful.

Fact: The need for specific types of assistive technology varies widely from one person to the next, but individuals of all ages, varying abilities and needs and all types of disabilities may be able to benefit from the use of technology.

Of course for every disabled person, there is a uniquely individual situation, which must not be discounted whether he or she decides to "learn new tricks." For it is a reality, that they must adjust to an environment in which disability is a constant, and they may never do things in exactly the same way they did them before.

CONCLUSION

Despite the limitations of having a disability, the elderly don't have to be saddled by the burden of a proverb that is far from being universally true. "Old dogs" can be taught and can learn "new tricks." The elderly disabled do not have to settle for a life that is moribund because of their disability. But to learn the new tricks that it will take to adjust to the challenging world configured by their disability they must have needed information about available resources; assistance in remedying transportation/mobility problems; an inner strength to overcome apathy; and be receptive to learning the benefits of change and assistive technology.

AUTHOR NOTE

With an extensive background in disability and human rights issues, Roger D. Ford is a former program manager for the community affairs and outreach branch of the D.C. Department of Human Rights and Minority Business Development. A certified rehabilitation counselor, Mr. Ford has worked with all disabilities in the capacity of teacher, counselor, social worker, and program manager. He is a graduate of Fisk University with a degree in chemistry and holds a master's degree in education and rehabilitation counseling from The George Washington University.

A former daily newspaper reporter in Charlotte, N.C., Janice E. Smith's articles have appeared in local Washington, D.C. publications as well as in national publications. She previously served as Associate Director for Information Services of the D.C. Department of Human Rights and Minority Business Development. A graduate of North Carolina A&T State University with a degree in English, she received her master's degree in journalism from The Ohio State University.

REFERENCES

Assistive Technology: Practical Intervention Strategies Handbook. (1993). District of Columbia Partnership for Assistive Technology (pp. 7-28).

Atkins, B.J., Ph.D., C.R.C. (1988). Rehabilitating Black Americans who are disabled. In S. Walker et al. *Building Bridges to Independence; Proceedings of the National Conference, Employment Successes, Problems and Needs of Black Americans with Disabilities.* Washington, D.C. (pp. 133; 137-138).

Bowe, F. (1985). Black adults with disabilities. A statistical report drawn from Census Bureau data.

B., C. (1994). Interview, D.C. Center for Independent Living, Washington, D.C.

Cott, C. and Wilkins, S. (1993). Aging, chronic illness and disability. In M. Nagler (Ed.), *Perspectives on Disability* (pp. 367, 368), Palo Alto, CA: Health Markets Research.

Galiber, Y.W. (1988). Vital links in the rehabilitation and employment of Black Americans with disabilities, a response. In S. Walker et al. *Building Bridges to Independence; Proceedings of the National Conference, Employment Successes, Problems and Needs of Black Americans with Disabilities.* Washington, D.C. (p. 177).

Green, R. (1992). Issues on crime, drugs, abuse and exploitation of the elderly in the District of Columbia. *Mayor's Conference on Aging: A Call to Action–The Future is Now.* Washington, D.C.(pp. 1–2).

P., O. (1994). Interview, D.C. Center for Independent Living, Washington, D.C.

P., B. (1994). Interview, D.C. Center for Independent Living, Washington, D.C.

Wilson, M.E., Jr., Ph.D. (1988). Critical factors in the employment success of Black Americans with Disabilities. In S. Walker et al. *Building Bridges to Independence; Proceedings of the National Conference, Employment Successes, Problems and Needs of Black Americans with Disabilities.* Washington, D.C.(p. 34).

Wright, B.A. (1983). Physical Disability–A Psychological Approach. (p. 236), New York: Harper & Row.

Wright, T.J., Ph.D., and Leung, P., Ph.D. (1993). Meeting the unique needs of minorities with disabilities. *A Report to the President and the Congress,* National Council on Disability, Washington, D.C. (p.14).

PART IV

LIFE EVENTS
AND SPIRITUALITY

Chapter 7

Keep the Faith:
A Biblical Reference to Surviving
the Social Transitions of Life

Ladd G. Colston

SUMMARY. The axiom "Keep the Faith" is addressed as a coping mechanism for surviving the social transitions of life. Leisure as a lifelong philosophy is applied as a conduit for daily reference of this religious phrase. Seven social transitions are discussed which are employed as adjustments to life events (i.e., death of spouse, illness and disability). Primarily found in later life, the stress of life events is documented as a major influence on the aging process. The role of religion and faith are found to be critical elements in one's personal adaptation to aging as well as surviving the uncertainty of life events. Religious phrases can be used to counsel individuals through problems and/or situations. The biblical reference "Keep the Faith" has direct links to faith in a supreme being and the belief that one can find a purpose for living and a means of coping with the unknown. Leisure activity is explored as a method of crisis intervention and a lifelong diet of nurturing emotions is recommended for well-being.

Words of encouragement can be used to empower individuals through the "bad times" and can be reinstated to celebrate the

Ladd G. Colston, PhD, is Associate Professor and Program Coordinator of Recreation and Leisure Studies, Department of HPER, Old Dominion University, Norfolk, VA 23529.

[Haworth co-indexing entry note]: "Keep the Faith: A Biblical Reference to Surviving the Social Transitions of Life." Colston, Ladd G. Co-published simultaneously in *Activities, Adaptation & Aging* (The Haworth Press, Inc.) Vol. 19, No. 2, 1994, pp. 75-85; and: *Aging Families and Use of Proverbs for Values Enrichment* (ed: Vera R. Jackson) The Haworth Press, Inc., 1994, pp. 75-85. Multiple copies of this article/chapter may be purchased from The Haworth Document Delivery Center [1-800-3-HA-WORTH; 9:00 a.m. - 5:00 p.m. (EST)].

occurrence of "good times." From generation to generation, inspirational words have been passed down in the form of common phrases or "sayings." Many of these phrases can be found to have a religious foundation or reference to them. Since mankind still has no rational explanation as to why certain life events occur unexpectantly (i.e., a tornado destroying a longstanding family home or a healthy friend suddenly contracting a terminal disease), there is a need to believe someone or something is in control, socially and/or spiritually. From natural disasters to man-made accidents and from unanticipated job opportunities to casually meeting one's future spouse, life events are an enigma within the life cycle. The uncertainty of these life events often creates a scenario of hope or despair. The former can evolve into a spiritual optimism where there is a sense of personal control; whereas, the latter reflects a pessimistic view of life that results in loss of control, futility and lastly, depression.

The life cycle is defined as a series of life stages which begin at birth and end at death. Each life stage brings behavioral change whether it is physical, mental, emotional, social or spiritual. Erik Erickson (1963) referred to these developmental life stages as a series of psycho-social crises which contribute to personality formation. He identified these crises as the eight (8) stages of Man. In stage eight (the crisis of ego integrity vs. despair), the individual searches for identity and self-acceptance as he/she prepares for the inescapable reality of death. Unresolved issues or crises in the individual's life make this stage a very critical one psychologically. From a phenomenological viewpoint, Erikson (1986) at age 87 expanded his perception of old age to reflect wisdom. He stated that "In old age, the struggle is between a sense of one's own integrity and a feeling of defeat, of despair about one's life in the phase of normal physical disintegration . . . the fruit of that struggle is wisdom." Successfully surviving the uncertainty of life events and understanding their complexity within the stages of life develops into an applied knowledge of the past which in turn can be passed down from generation to generation. One way in which this wisdom is transferred is through the axiom of "Keep the Faith." In this context, "faith" becomes the belief that one can and will successfully survive the social transitions of life. In faith, one can find a purpose for living and a means of coping with life events.

The role of religion in day to day living is a social phenomena that is characteristic of most communities throughout the world. Religion is found to be a critical element in one's personal adjustment to aging and surviving the uncertainty of life events (Moberg, 1989; Oyedeji, 1992; and van Manen, 1985). From this religious foundation, one can often find references to religious phrases that can be used to counsel individuals through problems and/or situations. One purpose of a person reading or reciting a religious phrase may be to bring hope that a positive blessing will occur that will in turn "get one through the day." The biblical reference "Keep the Faith" has direct links to faith in God and the belief that all will be made well in the end.

The aging process is an accumulation of behavioral changes that reflect a person's adjustment to social transitions occurring from life events. In brief, this process varies from person to person, from cohort to cohort and from culture to culture. Age is often defined in three ways: chronologically, experientially, and functionally. First, chronological age is fixed and progresses equally for all people. Second, experiential age refers to "age norms" that are implied by social responses such as "act your age." This definition refers to social behavior as projected by society which coincides with (1) a disengagement from certain activities (Cummings and Henry, 1961) and (2) an adoption of society's rules governing age appropriate behavior. Lastly, functional age is defined as an interrelationship of six factors: (1) tradition/culture and environment, (2) body or physical functioning, (3) mind or mental functioning, (4) self-concept, (5) occupation/avocation, and (6) stress. Contrary to the other two definitions, functional age implies an individualized approach to aging which adopts a developmental perspective. In this definition, the aging process builds upon a foundation of genetics and past experiences which in turn forms a foundation for the future. According to MacNeil and Teague (1987), leisure represents a lifelong learning philosophy of continuity and change. The ability to pursue familiar activities yet learn new activities builds upon the idea that every human being's life is a continuum. This lifespan approach to age and the application of leisure offers a means of crisis intervention for surviving the social transitions of life and referencing the phrase "Keep the Faith."

THE SOCIAL TRANSITIONS OF LIFE

Holmes and Rahe (1967) developed a stress test that encompassed a series of forty-three stressors listed as life events. The more significant the life event, the higher the stress. Each life event was given a number to reflect its impact on a person emotionally. The purpose of this test was to show how numerous stress producing events in a given time period put "wear and tear" on one's body, mind and spirit. Many of the most stressful life events that occur in Holmes and Rahe's stress test occur during times of social transition. In life, social transitions reflect human adaptations to change which are forced by unexplained life events. For this paper, seven social transitions will be discussed. They are as follows: (1) retirement, (2) subsistence reversal, (3) loss of spouse, (4) remarriage, (5) illness and disability, (6) institutionalized or residence relocation, and (7) new affiliations.

Retirement

Retirement is considered to be the single most significant modification determined by age. It is primarily guided by mass policy (i.e., the federal government at age 65) although ideally, retirement policies should be made on an individual basis. Unfortunately, retirement policies have often been used to force individuals out of work. For some, the results of forced retirement have produced a loss of identity, status, independence and financial security. For others, retirement can create a feeling of uselessness and boredom. If one is unable to adapt to this social transition, symptoms of depression can begin to surface.

The phrase "Keep the Faith" can be used to create alternatives to work and the absence of socializing with fellow employees. One means for transferring learned skills and experiences into new directions is through leisure activity participation. Leisure, referred to in later life as the second career (Colston, 1985), can be looked upon as a means of finding new challenges and providing a highly satisfying lifestyle. Work skills can be adapted into pleasurable forms of activity where vocational interests can become avocations of fun, pleasure and income. Numerous retirees have taken past skills, talents and knowledge and developed new businesses, specialized services or entered into consulting contracts.

Subsistence Reversal

The loss of autonomy and a transfer of personal power to a spouse, children or others connotates a major change for persons who were once called "bread winners." In many families, the husband or head of household was traditionally the major source of income and everyone was dependent upon what he could provide. Inadequate retirement income and other depleting resources can lead to a transferral of dependency onto others in order to provide support. In effect, the provider becomes the helpee. For many individuals, guilt develops and there is a major loss of self-worth and self-esteem.

A means of adjusting to this reversal and modification of social roles, with dignity intact, is critical for the individual involved. The role of provider or head of household can be redefined to include roles other than "bread winner." Family members can be asked to seek advice from the individual involved on such important matters as travel plans, shopping strategies and investments. Social visits to extended family members and friends can reinforce this new social role through leisure activity participation such as picnics, active sports and table games.

Loss of Spouse

Death of a spouse is most damaging to the survivor, especially if the relationship was happy. The loss of a spouse represents emotional turmoil that entails interpersonal relationships with children, brothers and sisters-in-law, friends and constituents. Legal problems regarding the "Will" and death benefits can result in strained relationships which were never intended but may go unresolved for years to come. The survivor takes on the personal burden of grief as well as the social encumbrance of loneliness and sorrow.

Mental and physical release is critical for establishing personal control during the social transition. "Keeping the Faith" that death is a part of life and the living must go on is a realization that a loss needs to be replaced with an acquisition. Leisure activity participation can be employed for developing new social contacts for companionship. Traveling abroad or becoming a member of a social club can be very instrumental in the overall maintenance of a satisfying life.

Remarriage

Finding another spouse can affect current and past relationships. Remarriage represents new social roles that can have a major impact on children and family from a previous marriage. Their acceptance and/or adjustment to the new spouse can have a strong bearing upon how the person is viewed and valued in the future. A father or mother can be encouraged to remarry or can be burdened with the guilt that the timing of this social transition is unacceptable. Past relationships can be strengthened or severed depending upon the impact of the remarriage. Those intimately involved may be forced to adjust to a new identity that may not be socially approved. In addition to significant others, the two persons involved in the remarriage will have to adjust to a new give and take relationship with themselves.

Leisure can be looked upon as a means of developing or finding mutuality, common values and security with one another. It can also be used as a means of introducing a potential suitor to family members in a non-threatening environment. A game of tennis, a fishing trip or a concert can be an ideal "ice-breaker" for developing interpersonal communications, mutual interests and acceptance with children from a previous marriage.

Illness and Disability

Two of the most limiting factors of life are illness and disability. Both impose restrictions that prevent full participation in activities of daily living. In addition, they limit the level of functional independence and frequency of participation that one may have grown accustomed to having in life. Psychological well-being is critical to one's survival of this social transition. The desire to continue living with the illness and/or disability must be established within the individual. Once there is evidence that the individual is willing to go on in life, then efforts can be exerted to rehabilitate the individual through activity modifications and learning new skills.

"Keep the Faith" has often been employed by family and friends at a sick bed or within the confines of a healthcare setting. One means of gaining limited, but functional independence is through leisure activity participation. Community involvement and social interaction can become realistic goals for the individual. For one to participate in recreational (leisure) activity, one should possess interest (intrinsic motivation) and have access to opportunity (freedom). Assistive technology, therapeutic recreation and/or activity therapy are service mechanisms that can facilitate behavior change, skill acquisition, leisure education and resource referral (i.e., water walking for muscle strength and endurance; gardening–horticultural therapy–for developing fine motor dexterity).

Institutionalization or Residence Relocation

Relocation from a familiar environment such as a home of twenty-five years represents a loss of environmental control. This loss creates a situation where a person is forced to relinquish self-determination, especially in a nursing facility where one is governed by the policies and procedures of the institution. Moving in with a family member also represents environmental change. Moves are usually traumatic and require great sensitivity by those involved. Even in a senior living facility where residents can still lead active lives, compatibility with neighbors and services must be successfully implemented if one is to adapt to this social transition.

Leisure can be looked upon as a means of assisting a new resident or patient with exerting some control over life choices within a restricted environment. Resident-run advisory groups and newsletters can provide assurances that one's voice can be heard in a retirement community. Current legislation and legal statutes are designed to ensure "quality of life" leisure-based activities for consumers of nursing facilities. Traditional family activities can be periodically instituted to provide stability and input by the relocated family member. "Keep the faith" is symbolic of change, a change that through leisure can reverse a powerless situation into an empowering experience.

New Affiliations

Often times, relocating to a new environment results in a loss of social group, peers, friends and/or community involvements. New affiliations may require social contacts or a need to (re)develop interpersonal communication skills. If assistance is not made available, one can easily find themselves in isolation and on the verge of depression. Life satisfaction is integral to surviving these transitions.

The American Association for Retired Persons (AARP) and community-based senior centers currently offer opportunities for developing new peer relationships. Enrolling in a community college class, observing available recreation/social programs and/or volunteering at a local hospital can provide additional access to new social contacts. "Keep the faith" acknowledges that everybody needs somebody sometimes and that no man or woman can remain "an island in the sea of life." Leisure activities can facilitate social interaction, new activity interests and active participation. Leisure service providers can also be instrumental in introducing a new community member to a social group, organization or compatible peer. New affiliations are crucial to one's adjustment to the loss of past affiliations, whether through relocation or death.

LEISURE AND LIFE SATISFACTION

Life satisfaction is defined as a cognitive assessment of one's progress toward one's desired goals in life. Life satisfaction is integral to surviving these seven social transitions and leisure is a viable tool that can be applied to each one. Research has shown that lifestyle habits are integral to longevity and a better quality of life (O'Brien and Vertinsky, 1991). The American Medical Association has observed that 8 out of the top 10 major causes of death in the United States are related to smoking, diet and alcohol abuse. Quality of life has become a central theme in healthcare and has been found to be a function of physical and psychological well-being.

Iso-Ahola and Weisinger (1984) found that socialization into satisfying leisure experiences and behaviors throughout childhood and adolescence are likely to form the foundation for the "intrinsic motivation predisposition." This personality trait protects people form stress and consists of three components: (1) commitment, (2) challenge, and (3) control. The axiom "Keep the Faith" makes reference to the future and the lifelong philosophy of leisure lends credence to its usefulness as an incentive for living. A positive approach to enhancing life satisfaction in later life can be the ability to nurture emotions for well-being. Burdman (1986) made reference to an emotional diet that was offered by Helen Ansley, an octogenarian who provided an interesting perspective to seeking joy in later life. Ms. Ashley's diet was comprised of the five A's: (1) acceptance (the need to belong and associate with others whose aims and values are similar to our own), (2) appreciation (the need to feel needed and a recognition of the value of difference), (3) affection (the need to feel concern for someone other than ourselves and to recognize that the happiness of other people is important), (4) achievement (the need to feel that we accomplished something by our efforts), and (5) amusement (the need for laughter, fun and games). Since the ups and downs of ordinary daily life provide a mixed diet of emotions, Ms. Ashley referenced emotions to avoid. These emotions were fear, frustration, inferiority and guilt. The latter emotion (guilt) can elicit remorse and promote depression.

Krause and Van-Tran (1989) found that although life stress tends to erode feelings of self-worth and mastery, these negative effects can be offset or counterbalanced by increased religious involvement. Aging must be viewed as a process and an opportunity for growth and enlightenment. The biblical reference "Keep the Faith" implies that there are better days ahead and that persons who are believers can survive the social transitions of life.

REFERENCES

Bandura, A. (1977). A Social Learning Theory. Englewood Cliffs, New Jersey: Prentice-Hall, Inc.
Bergin, Allen E. (1989). Religious faith and counseling: A commentary on Worthington. *Counseling Psychologist*, Vol. 17 (4), pp. 621-623.

Burdman, Geri Marr. (1986). Healthful aging. Englewood Cliffs, New Jersey: Prentice Hall, Inc.

Caspi, Avshalom. (1987). Personality in the life course. Special Issue: Integrating personality and social psychology. *Journal of Personality and Social Psychology*, Vol. 53 (6), pp. 1203-1213.

Chipperfield, Judith. (1993). Perceived barriers in coping with health problems : A twelve-year longitudinal study of survival among elderly individuals. *Journal of Aging and Health*, Vol. 5 (1), pp. 123-139.

Colston, Ladd. (1986). Leisure and aging: An incentive for living. *Parks and Recreation*, Vol 21 (8), pp. 35-42.

Cummings, Elaine and Henry, W.E. (1961). *Growing Old: The Process of Disengagement*. New York: Basic Books.

Dychtwald, Ken and Flower, Joe. (1989). *Age Wave: The Challenges and Opportunities of an Aging America*. Los Angeles, California: Jeremy P. Tarcher, Inc.

Erickson, Eric. (1963). *Childhood and Society*. New York: W.W. Norton and Company, Inc.

Erickson, Erik, Erickson, Joan and Kivnick, Helen. (1986). *Vital Involvement in Old Age*. New York: W. W. Norton and Company, Inc.

Fletcher, Wesla and Hansson, Robert. (1991). Assessing the social components of retirement anxiety. *Psychology and Aging*, Vol. 6 (1), pp. 76-85.

Holmes, Thomas and Rahe, Robert. (1967). The Social readjustment rating scale. *Journal of Psychosomatic Research*, Vol. 11, pp. 213-218.

Howe, Christine. (1987). Selected social gerontology theories and older adult leisure involvement: A review of the literature. *The Journal of Applied Gerontology*, Vol. 6(4), pp. 448-463.

Iso-Aholo, Seppo and Weissinger, Ellen. (1984). Leisure and well being: Is there a connection? *Parks and Recreation*, Vol. 9 (6), pp. 40-43.

Krause, Neal and Van-Tran, Thanh. (1989). Stress and religious involvement among older Blacks. *Journal of Gerontology*, Vol. 44 (1), pp. S4-S13.

Lavee, Yoav; McCubbin, Hamilton and Olson, David. (1987). The effect of stressful life events and transitions on family functioning and well-being. *Journal of Marriage and the Family*, Vol. 49 (4), pp. 857-873.

Leitner, Michael and Leitner, Sara. (1985). *Leisure in Later Life: A Sourcebook for the Provision of Recreational Services for Elders*. New York, NY: The Haworth Press, Inc.

MacNeil, Richard and Teague, Michael. (1987). *Aging and Leisure: Vitality in later Life* Englewood Cliffs, New Jersey: Prentice-Hall, Inc.

McCandless, J. Bardarah. (1991). The church confronting adult depression: A challenge. Special Issue: Depression and religion. *Counseling and Values Vol. 35 (92), pp. 104-113*.

Moberg, David. (1989). Religion and personal adjustment in old age: A replication and explication. Paper presented at the Annual Meeting of the Gerontological Society of America, 42nd, Minneapolis, MN, November 17-21, (1989), 24 pp.

Neugarten, Bernice. (1979). Time, age and the life cycle. *American Journal of Psychiatry,* Vol. 136 no. 7, pp. 887-894.

O'Brien, Sandra and Vertinsky, Patricia. (1991). Unfit survivors: Exercise as a resource for aging women. *Gerontologist,* Vol. 31 (3), pp. 347-357.

Payne, Christopher; Robbins, Steven and Dougherty, Linda. (1991). Goal directedness and older adult adjustment. *Journal of Counseling Psychology,* Vol. 38 (93), pp. 302-308

Thomas, Carolyn and Martin, Virginia. (1992). Training counselors to facilitate the transitions of aging through group work. Special section: Training in gerontological counseling. *Counselor Education and Supervision,* Vol. 32 (1), pp. 51-60.

Chapter 8

Faith of our Fathers (Mothers) Living Still: Spirituality as a Force for the Transmission of Family Values Within the Black Community

Joseph Dancy, Jr.
M. Lorraine Wynn-Dancy

SUMMARY. This paper examines spirituality as a focus for the Black elderly's transmission of family values within the Black community. The process of aging is presented as a spiritual journey which offers the elderly opportunity for continued growth. The grandparents' roles in transmitting values through the oral tradition of story telling and proverbs remains significant within the Black community, though urban crowding has diminished their influence in more recent decades. Strengths of the Black elderly in coping with life's vicissitudes are demonstrated through their proverbs with messages of faith and hope.

Joseph Dancy, Jr., PhD, is Gerontologist/Associate Professor in the Ethelyn R. Strong School of Social Work at Norfolk State University in Norfolk, VA.

M. Lorraine Wynn-Dancy, MS, MA, is currently Assistant Professor and Program Director in the Department of Community Health and Rehabilitation at Norfolk State University in Norfolk, VA.

Address correspondence to: 1501 Hadley Court, Virginia Beach, VA 23456

[Haworth co-indexing entry note]: "Faith of Our Fathers (Mothers) Living Still: Spirituality as a Force for the Transmission of Family Values Within the Black Community." Dancy, Joseph Jr., and M. Lorraine Wynn-Dancy. Co-published simultaneously in *Activities, Adaptation & Aging* (The Haworth Press, Inc.) Vol. 19, No. 2, 1994, pp. 87-105; and: *Aging Families and Use of Proverbs for Values Enrichment* (ed: Vera R. Jackson) The Haworth Press, Inc., 1994, pp. 87-105. Multiple copies of this article/chapter may be purchased from The Haworth Document Delivery Center [1-800-3-HAWORTH; 9:00 a.m. - 5:00 p.m. (EST)].

INTRODUCTION

Perhaps few concepts in the field of gerontology are as exciting as the increasing regard that the process of aging can be viewed more as a spiritual journey than a biological one. C. S. Heriot (1992) in her article, "Spirituality and Aging" noted that researchers have proposed that aging is a spiritual rather than biologic process.

> There is no evidence, however, that the spirit succumbs to the aging process, even in the presence of debilitating physical and mental illness . . . (Philibert, 1981) also said that aging as a spiritual growth is an opportunity that may be enjoyed or neglected. (Heriot, 1992)

This assertion is affirmed by Moberg (1971) who noted that in later life it is matters of the spirit that offer the greatest opportunity for continued growth. He stated that the human domain "that stands out as providing the most opportunity for continued growth in the latter years is the spiritual" (Moberg, p. 30).

Considering these researchers' findings, it becomes apparent that the elderly are special repositories of each culture's spiritual values. This is especially true for the Black elderly.

In the transmission of family values within the traditional Black community the Black elderly are the pivotal axis. Joseph White (1984) in his work, *The Psychology of Blacks: An Afro-American Perspective*, penned these observations:

> Older people in the Black community are the reservoirs of the wisdom accumulated during the experiences of a life time. They are the storehouses of the oral tradition and the keepers of the heritage.
>
> The elderly are valued because they have been through the experiences that can only come with age. They have been 'down the line,' as the saying goes, seen the comings and goings of life, and been through the repetitive cycles of oppression, struggle, survival, backlash, and renewed struggle. Older people have stood the test of time and adversity, paid their dues, transcended tragedy, and learned how to keep on keepin' on. (White, 1984, p. 44)

Spirituality is deeply rooted in the Black psyche (Knox, 1985). This strong sense of spirituality has its roots in African religious traditions (Mbiti, 1969 and Nobles, 1980). Religion and religious institutions are quite pivotal in the Black community with the Black elderly particularly attached to these institutions. Only the family ranks as more important in the Black community than the church (Taylor, 1986).

Moberg (1971) has put forth the definition of religion as "the personal beliefs, values, and activities pertinent to that which is supernatural, mysterious and awesome, which transcends immediate situations and which pertains to questions of final causes and ultimate ends of man and the universe." In their article, "Religion and Well-Being in Later Life" in *The Gerontologist*, Harold G. Koening, James N. Kvale et al. (1988) report Moberg as pointing out two basic orientations of religion: personal and institutional. While the institutional orientation focuses on group-related behaviors such as church attendance and organizational religious rituals, personal religious orientation reflects individual values, beliefs and attitudes. Prayer and reading of devotional literature are within the realm of personal religious orientation. It is of interest to note that these authors comment that "personal religious attitudes and private devotional activities may be more relevant indicators of religiosity for aged individuals" (Koenig et al., 1988). Frankl (1978) has also emphasized that the spirit is the distinction which separates humans from animals, thus making the spirit the most fundamental unit of being human.

It is important to observe in this discussion of spirituality among the Black elderly that spirituality is more encompassing than the term religion. In fact spirituality may be conceived as the umbrella concept under which one finds religion and the needs of the human spirit. Religion and spirituality are not synonymous. Religion refers to an external, formal system of beliefs, whereas spirituality is conceived more with a personal interpretation of life and the inner resources of people (Heriot, 1992, p. 23). Thus, 'spirituality' can be classified independently of 'religion.' In other words, spirituality's home may be within as well as outside the institutional church or organized religion. By contrast, it must be made clear that all facets of religion can not be assumed to be spiritual (C. K. Chandler et al., 1992).

Moberg (1971) has pointed out this observation:

> There is a distinction . . . between 'spiritual' and 'religious.' While not necessarily opposites, they are not synonymous. A spiritual need may be met by a religious act, such as praying or receiving Holy Communion, but many spiritual needs are met by warm and sympathetic human relationships. Often a spiritual need is best met by dealing with a physical need.
>
> To assume that everything 'religious' is therefore also 'spiritual' or vice versa is a serious fallacy. . . . The concepts overlap, but they are not synonymous. . . . The human spirit can be addressed both within and outside of the context of religion."

For the Black elderly, also, the spiritual dimension includes the development of some meaning for life. Attempts to understand suffering, as well as mitigation of forgiveness, fountains of love, relatedness and transcendence, as well as an inner experience of trust in God as the supreme Being are all part of the spiritual realm (Heriot, 1992, p. 23).

Ross (1981) has observed that "the spiritual resources of aging are the strengths and learnings gleamed from a life time of experiences." Having survived over 65 years of numerous disappointments, losses, and tragedies, the elderly will have "cultivated some know-how that will serve them in the last years of life" (Ross, 1981, p. 26).

The spiritual self is partially defined through interaction with others. Particularly in the latter stage of life, the spiritual self is viewed through introspection and contemplation. Older adults tend to be more likely to discard primary concerns centered on status within the working world and materialism. Rather interpersonal relationships take center stage. Certainly, a hallmark of this stage of the life cycle is the opportunity to think about spiritual matters. As death looms, issues such as mortality, immortality, love relationships, and transcendence may develop fresh or reinvigorated purport (Beck, 1984).

Maslow (1971) has declared that part of the human essence is spiritual life (the contemplative, religious, philosophical or value-life). He observed that spirituality is a defining characteristic of human nature.

Assagioli (1965) notes that 'spiritual' refers not only to experiences traditionally considered religious but to all the states of awareness, all the human functions and activities which have as their common denomination the possession of values higher than the average . . . spiritual drives or spiritual urges are . . . real, basic and fundamental" (Assagioli, 1965, p. 194).

The deepest requirements of the self are spiritual needs, asserts Moberg (1971), and the meeting of spiritual needs allows a person to function with a meaningful identity and purpose. Thus, an individual proceeds through the stages of life with reality fortified by hope.

Though several definitions of the spiritual abound, Moberg (1971) adds the following:

> It (spirituality) is variously interpreted as the realm of faith, revelation, illumination, and insight, in contrast to the realm of phenomena which are empirically observable by man through his senses. The spiritual represents the totality of commitment—the total man-God relationship which sensory experiences reflect only in part.

For the elderly, as well, spirituality focuses on man's "ultimate concern." The spiritual realm provides meaning to matters within a culture. The totality of human value orientation is included. In fact, the spiritual realm goes beyond a culture's religious beliefs and practices when these become "frozen into rigid traditional forms, and (the spiritual realm) is not recognized by those who seek religion only in churches (Moberg, 1971).

The theologian, Howard Thurman (1963) has mused that man is more than body, more than mind and more than spirit. The totality of man incorporates the spirit, and in man's spirit there is the crucial nexus that links him with Creator of Life.

The spiritual, thus, can be viewed as "the basic value around which all other values are focused, the central philosophy of life . . . which guides a person's conduct, the supernatural and nonmaterial dimensions of human nature. We assure that men are spiritual even if they have no use for religious institutions and practice no personal pieties" (Moberg, 1971).

It is against this theological/anthropological backdrop that one can attest to the important role of the Black elderly in transmission of family values within the Black community through their spirituality. Dancy (1977) noted the religious experience of the Black elderly remains a unique aspect of the Black cultural experience. With a strong orientation toward religion, the Black church has a significant and endeared place in the lives of many Black elderly. Their religion has been an anchor when oppressive forces have heaved against their lives. Religion and the Black church have thrown life lines to the Black elderly to provide them hope for survival and advancement in an often threatening climate within the larger community.

"The religious experience of the Black elderly, especially those from the low income group, helps them to value life. They do not fear death (in a religious sense) because of the hope they hold for life after death" (Dancy, 1977, p. 23).

In her work, *Black Families in Therapy*, Nancy Boyd-Franklin (1989) also comments that religion and spirituality are important aspects of the strengths and coping skills Black families call upon to transverse life's journey. Though all Blacks are not members of organized religions or churches, many have a well-developed internal sense of spirituality.

Other researchers including Billingsley (1968) and Hill (1971) have stressed the well-documented fact that religion and the church are important vestiges for the Black family. Aging persons appear to especially find religion of increasing importance, and religion appears to be of particular significance to a large percentage of the Black elderly (Heisel et al., 1982).

TRANSMISSION OF FAMILY VALUES

It should be clear from the discussion thus far that spirituality of some form is a part of every human's basic needs. Just how does spirituality or any value get transmitted to the young within a society? Certainly, a society's elders play a key role in any value transference within the Black community.

The elderly are also an important reservoir for the transmission of family values. Aunts, uncles, older cousins and, especially grandparents, are vital links to deeply held values within the Black community.

Barrow (1992) has observed that more frequently communities have three-generation families, and that four and five generation families are on the rise. More than seventy percent of older persons have grandchildren, and at least fifty percent have great-grandchildren.

An important question for continued investigation is whether the Black elderly act as mediators between the Black child and society as the child develops his sense of self-worth and value (Nobles, 1987) noted:

> Within these Black families, the elderly hold a special position. They represent the keepers of the family's history and, accordingly, have been given respect for their insights and guidance in matters of the family. Story-telling is used as a means of transmitting a particular culture to the young in Black families. The elderly are most often the storytellers in the family, thereby serving the critical function of instilling in the young, via the stories, a sense of history and a sense of a family.

Thus, the Black elderly are vital to the process of transmitting values within Black communities and spiritual values are certainly among those being transmitted. Beaver (1990) has emphasized that the family, friends, benevolent societies and church have been significant in assuaging Blacks' humiliation with slavery and its residuals. He observes that "as it did during slavery, the church continues to play an important role in the lives of Black people, particularly old Blacks. A strong interdependence among generations also developed . . . intensive patterns of kinship interaction have survived among Black people" (Beaver, 1990).

In the discussion of the transmission of spiritual values by Black elders, it is important to reflect briefly as to just what is meant by values. O'Driscoll (1976) has observed that "values denote an evaluative representation of a person or group's perception of his/her or their relationship to the social/physical environments." Borsodi

(1965) gives the reminder that values are reflected in every human action and that each human institution is an outgrowth of a social value. Sperry (1974) agrees with Borsodi's assertion when he states that "human values stand out as a universal determinant of all human decisions and activities" (Sperry, 1974, p. 9).

With the awareness of the universality of value lines in every culture, it is necessary, even crucial, to be cognizant as to the purveyors of value in the Black community. Traditionally, the Black elderly have had a pivotal role and their spiritual values have permeated many Black communities.

V. Robert Hayles (1991), based on the work of Cook and Kono (1977), observes that "African American value systems can be summarized by pointing to their emphasis on harmony and rhythm; soul and internal development or consciousness" (Hayles, 1991, p. 314). V. Robert Hayles (1991) has pointed out that empirically documented strengths of Black families include value systems that nurture harmony, cooperation, interdependence, acceptance of difference, internal development, strong work/achievement orientation and traditionalism. Certainly, the Black elders are crucial in the transmitting of these values. In fact, Hayles (1991) continues by stressing that the respect, appreciation and full utilization of the skills and wisdom of senior family members is a strength of Black families.

Hill (1971) has also cited cultural themes which have bolstered Black families during critical times. In addition to strong kinship bonds among varied households, much flexibility in family roles and high work, education and achievement orientation, Hill notes that a strong commitment to religious values and church participation also emerges as a cultural theme in Black families.

The discussion of how values are transmitted appears incomplete without centralizing values within a culture. A necessary detail is pointing out that values are only one aspect of the jigsaw puzzle called culture. Culture incorporates values, ideas, concepts and expected behaviors (Brislin, 1993). Thus, in highlighting spiritual values and the Black elderly's important role, it must be borne in mind that this is a minuscule, though dominant, feature in the umbrella called culture within any given Black community.

R. R. Greene (1986) cautions that "culture is produced by persons who live in it" (Greene, 1986, p. 127). This writer then points to Taylor (1974) who noted culture is that complex whole which includes knowledge, beliefs, art, morals, laws, customs and any other capabilities and habits acquired by man as a member of society.

Green (1986) then adds this illumination:

> Every individual is a product of a particular culture, created by a particular society or group that gives him/her a road map for living; every family is also a product of the general culture and in addition every family develops a culture of its own. Culture influences a person's world view, understanding, actions and feelings. It shapes each person's social recognition, connectedness, and aspiration toward self-realization. The family as a primary and universal human group, helps maintain the culture. (Greene, 1986, p. 127-128)

> Cultures shape the cycle of growth of its members. Within the context of its culture, the family maintains itself throughout its life by adhering to its own particular values, which are a conception, explicit or implicit, distinctive of an individual or characteristic of a group, of that which is desirable. (Greene, 1986, p. 128)

Indeed, it is a family's value system that impacts the life and activity of a family in the movement from one developmental task to the next (Greene, 1986). Thus, it is within the context of the Black culture that the Black elderly's pivotal role in the transmission of spiritual values must be viewed.

Brislin (1993) has commented on the length of time it takes for a particular value to become focal in any society. He also states that cultural values exist for lengthy periods once rooted in a society with examples of values reflected in the oral and written literature of a culture. " . . . cultural values cannot be introduced quickly. It usually takes years for people to become familiar enough with a new value or ideal for it to be considered part of their culture" (Brislin, 1993, p. 6).

Thus, the impact of the Black elderly's transmission of spiritual values to the young within the Black community represents generations of spiritual traditions within the Black religious institutions.

What about urbanization? What impact has this phenomenon had on the Black elderly's status within the urban Black community, and hence, the ability of the Black elderly to transmit spiritual values to the young? Martin and Martin (1979) have observed that those living in urban centers have more difficulties than their rural kinsfolk in matters relating to raising and educating their children and keeping them out of trouble. They offer the insight that one reason for this possible negative fallout from urban life is:

> the diminished role of the aged. Housing patterns tend to squeeze the aged out of urban extended families. The aged are not as available as they are in rural areas to babysit, for working parents, to informally adopt children, and to teach children religious values, respect for hard work, respect for authority, the importance of education, the difference between right and wrong, and so on. Children's socialization in the city is largely influenced by peer groups, the streets, the mass media and the schools. (p. 164)

Martin and Martin's words of caution about the impact of urbanization on Black family life, and the reduced role of urban Black elders as the purveyors of the culture's values, including possibly spiritual values can be lamented. Though the diminished role of elders within large urban corridors has been recorded, there remain countless hamlets, villages, small towns and large towns where Black elders have remained welcome, available and willing to nurture their community's young, including providing the youth with ready access to the Black culture's spiritual values.

ROLE OF GRANDPARENTS
AND THE ORAL TRADITION OF VALUES

C. S. Kart (1994) has indicated among the elderly about seventy-five percent have living grandchildren. In fact, about fifty percent of grandparents in the United States see a grandchild practically every day.

On the five styles of grandparenting delineated by Neugarten and Weinstein (1964), it is the style of the "grandparent as the reservoir of family wisdom" which is of particular interest to this discussion. When grandparents assume the role of reservoirs they are believed to have special skills and resources that younger parents need. The grandparents designated as reservoirs also expect younger parents to allow the elders to maintain a more dominant position in family life.

The prominent role of the oral tradition within the Black community has provided grandparents with a ready means for ease of value transmission. Grandparents who are reservoirs are ever ready with a story from the past, including biblical stories, that emphasize a value or trait the young will need along life's journey.

Brislin (1993) highlighted the elders' role with the young in the transmission of values:

> . . . values considered central to a society that have existed for many years . . . must be transmitted from one generation to another. Children must learn the values from various elders who have the responsibility to make sure that the children grow up to be acceptable members of the community. These elders include the children's parents, teachers, note worthy community figures, such as politicians and physicians, religious leaders, and so forth . . . (Brislin, 1993, p. 6-7)

Howard (1991) also stressed the importance of the elders' stories in teaching the children in a culture guidance about proper behavior.

Mary Frances Berry, and John Blassingame (1982) have examined the elders' role during the post emancipation period. They note that in spite of the lack of time, intensely religious parents taught moral lessons to their children by example. "They inculcated respect for elders and the dignity of work and stressed the importance of obtaining property and of education" (Berry et al., 1982, p. 79).

There are few young Blacks who have been in frequent contact with grandparents with strong spiritual and moral values who have not confided to their parents and friends that grandmother or grandfather has been "preaching" to them again. In other words, the grandparents have firmly lectured the young on what is good or bad behavior within their family, and expectations that the young Blacks would "toe the line" or do as expected in observing proper behavior. Biblical proverbs have often been utilized in these preachments.

Proverbs, especially, are of interest in examining the Black elderly's preachments and oral tradition. A proverb is a short, popular maxim that contains a moral or ethical truth. These epigrams become widely heard on the lips of all segments of a community. Such proverbial sayings generally originate and are given "long life" by the elderly in a community. Proverbial apothegms are cogent and instructive sayings that generally lack metaphorical qualities. However, the proverbial statements of particular interest in examining the oral traditions and spirituality of the Black elderly are biblical proverbs, such as these: "The Lord will make a way somehow"; "It's God's will"; "The Man upstairs will take care of it"; or "He won't give you more than you can bear."

The depth with which spiritual values are lodged within the bowels of the Black community can be contributed to the position of dominance and respect many Black elders traditionally held in the Black community. Many hamlets and small towns, especially, still revere the elders who often have been, also, long time leaders of the local church. While elders' advice, admonishments, proverbs and stories to youth are legendary in many Black communities, one would need to investigate more fully the impact of urban crowded housing on the more diminished influence of the Black elderly within inner urban corridors. Perhaps, the more open environmental spaces of smaller towns and cities allowed the Black elderly to remain influential to promote spiritual and other positive values, yet not "take up space" in an over-crowded urban apartment.

However, such spiritual values as faith and hope in a Higher Power are within the very core of most Black communities. The Black elders have left a profound spiritual legacy. Mitchell and Lewter (1986) noted that people who grow up in a traditional Black community are spontaneously equipped with a system of core beliefs, especially spiritual ones. Knox (1985) reports that one often hears these refrains in the Black community: "God will know what your needs are and will supply," and "He gives you no more than you can carry" (Knox, 1985, p. 2). Boyd-Franklin (1989) comments that these spiritual refrains underscore the "inner strength of the person and the power of this faith and belief system" (Boyd-Franklin, 1989, p. 79).

The idea of the extended family is a well-documented feature of Black family life. Not only grandparents but older aunts, uncles, cousins and even neighbors have often given advice to young Blacks to "show them the way." Thus, many spiritual values also get espoused outside the church as the elders communicate with the youth within the communities. Biblical references can be heard frequently within many homes in the Black community where references to the spiritual realm punctuate conversations. Some would say these spiritual values are "there in the air" because of the strongly held spiritual beliefs by many of the community's elders.

The importance of the extended family's role since post-emancipation days is shared by Berry and Blassingame (1982) when they stated that "after slavery the extended family was prevalent in the Black community. Generally, Black households had twice as many relatives outside the immediate family as did White ones. Egalitarian in nature, the family was marked by flexibility of roles, informal adoption of children and care of the aged" (Berry et al., 1982, p. 85).

A grandchild moving in to live with grandparents has been a common phenomenon throughout the documented history of the Black family from post-emancipation times to the present. Berry and Blassingame (1982) observed that "many autobiographers were reared by grandparents and other relatives. In spite of their own poverty, relatives enthusiastically tried to provide for orphaned children." Numerous famous Blacks attest to the fine rearing of grandparents as the significant difference in their going the "straight and narrow way." Frederick Douglass shared in his autobiography the love he felt for his grandmother and the profound impact she had on his early life in the slave quarters (Staples, 1986).

Staples (1986) has also pointed that those persons who informally adopt relatives are likely to be grandparents (or aunts or uncles). The historic fortitude and self-reliance of the Black elderly is vividly reflected in the fact that they are more likely to take others into their households than to be taken into the households of younger relatives (Staples, 1986, p. 197).

Special reference must be made to the Black grandmother as a purveyor of spiritual values with occasionally several generations residing within her household (Berry et al., 1982).

Certainly the Black grandmother frequently has considerable opportunity to impart spiritual values to her family due to her often ready proximity. Hill (1972) stated:

> In families headed by a woman, the Black families demonstrated an even greater tendency to absorb other related relatives. . . . But the families headed by elderly women take in the highest proportion (48%) of children. . . . These elderly persons play important roles in many of those families . . . with grandchildren. (Hill 1972, p. 5)

The centrality of the grandmother's role in Black family life is also observed by other researchers. This elder is lauded for her economic and nurturing support within Black families. Grandparent figures have been a "major source of strength and security for many Black children" (N.B. Franklin, 1989, p. 71). Boyd-Franklin (1989) goes on to state that the grandmother still has a powerful position in many extended Black families. "Often it is the grandmother who really makes the important decisions in a child's life . . . " (Boyd-Franklin, 1989, p. 73).

Thus, the grandparents often maintain a respected role within the family, and are able to play a significant role in shaping the spiritual values, as well as other values of the young. Jackson (1971) has also shared that "findings indicate that many Black grandparents serve as a point of anchorage for grandchildren and provide kinds of supports for them unavailable from their own parents" (Jackson, 1971, p. 193).

There is a sense in which the past is in every person. It is in every person in that which has been conveyed to individuals by their grandparents, thus, impacting their lives within the current times. A line from the hymn, "Faith of our Mothers," also reinforces this point:

> Faith of our mothers, living still, In cradle song and bedtime prayer; In nursery lore and fireside love, Thy presence still pervades the air.

Thus, the powerful positive presence and the beauty of the Black elders' spirits pervades today's air through stories, proverbs, scriptural passages and statements of spiritual value that the elders shared with today's adults during the latter's childhood. Consider the following examples that provide windows of light to the above point. Howard Thurman in his book tells this story:

> ... coming home from school,. ... a classmate began to bully me. I took all I could and then the fight was on. It was a hard and bitter fight. The fact that he was larger and older than I, and had brothers, did not matter. For four blocks we fought and there was no one to separate us. I got him to the ground and he conceded defeat. Then I had to come home to face my grandmother. "No one ever wins a fight," were her only words as she looked at me. "But I beat him," I said. "Yes, but look at yourself."

For Thurman and, no doubt others, the proverb "No one ever wins a fight," has become a lingering legacy from the past that resides in the being of today's adults.

Or consider the account of that adult father who shares in his own words his grandparents' value statement:

> Even if you want to be a trash man, *"strive to be the best one,"* my grandmother would say. My father taught me that I would achieve more in life if I treated people right, "Do unto others as you would have them do unto you," even if they didn't treat me right. I pass these themes (proverbs) on to my son.

Again, in his sharing and passing these themes or proverbs from his grandmother on to his son, the faith of his grandmother is living still.

Finally there is a biblical basis for the elders being a major reservoir for the transmission of our spiritual legacy to the young within the Black community. In Paul's letter to Timothy (II Timothy 1:5 RSV) he states: "I am reminded of your sincere faith, a faith that dwells first in your grandmother Lois and your mother Eunice and now, I am sure, dwells in you." To Timothy, his son in the ministry, Paul recalls that he is a debtor to the faith of his fathers, and shares with Timothy that he stands on the shoulders of at least the third generation of faith. For African Americans our spiritual legacy has continued the themes and proverbs of faith and hope. It has found, in part, expression in statements like these: The Lord will make a way somehow; The Lord will provide; Where there is a will, there is a way.

Some of the above proverbs, no doubt, have been imprinted on the hearts and minds of those who sat in the presence of the elders. Thurman said of the elders:

> They added to the security given to me by the quiet insistence of my mother and especially my grandmother that their children's lives were a precious gift . . . She (grandma) would gather us around and tell us a story that came from her life as a slave.

To that end the faith of our fathers (mothers) is living still.

CONCLUSION

This paper has examined spirituality as a conveyance of the Black elderly's values within the Black family and community. The process of aging is viewed as a spiritual journey which offers the elderly opportunity for continued growth. The distinction between spirituality and religion was clarified. Religion refers to an external, formal dogma incorporated in rituals within an institutional framework. However, spirituality is defined as a more encompassing term than religion with contemplation, personal prayer and a personal interpretation of life operative either within or outside the institutional church. The Black elderly demonstrate and appear strengthened by a strong orientation toward religion. The Black elderly are a major reservoir for the transmission of family values. In particular, Black elderly transmit spiritual values to the young within the Black community through the oral tradition utilizing stories and proverbs. It is suggested that urbanization may have diminished some of the Black elderly's influence on spiritual values because crowded urban conditions made the elderly less welcome in family households. With statistics indicating, however, that fifty percent of grandparents see a grandchild practically every day, grandparents remain significant figures as purveyors of spiritual values through proverbs and stories within the Black community with messages of faith and hope.

AUTHOR NOTE

Dr. Joseph Dancy, Jr. is a theologian/gerontologist. He received his undergraduate degree from Virginia Union University, the Master of Theology (ThM.) degree from Princeton Theological Seminary in Princeton, NJ, and the Doctor of Philosophy (PhD) degree in Educational Gerontology from the University of Michigan, Ann Arbor, MI. He is the author of the book, *The Black Elderly: A Guide for Practitioners* and co-authored the books, *Mature/Older Job Seeker's Guide* and *Health Promotion for the Rural Black Elderly: A Program Planning and Implementation Guide.*

M. Lorraine Wynn-Dancy received her undergraduate degree from Hampton University, a Master's degree (MS) in Speech and Hearing Science from Michigan State University and a Master's degree (MA) in Linguistics from The University of Michigan, Ann Arbor, MI. She has completed additional studies at the University of Nigeria, in Nussuka, Nigeria, West Africa and at Stanford University in Palo Alto, CA.

REFERENCES

Assagioli, R. (1965). *Psychosynthesis: A Manual of Principles and Techniques.* New York: Viking Penguin.

Barrow, G. M. (1992). *Aging the Individual and Society,* 5th ed. St. Paul, Minnesota: West Publishing Co.

Beaver, Marion. "The Older Person in the Black Family." In S. M. L. Logan, E. Freeman and R. McRoy, *Social Work Practice With Black Families: A Culturally Specific Perspective.* N.Y.: Longman Co., 1990.

Beck, C. M. (1984). "The Aged Adult." In C. M. Beck, R. P. Rawlins, S. R. Williams, eds., *Mental Health-Psychiatric Nursing: A Holistic Life-Cycle Approach.* St. Louis: Mosby Co.

Berry, M. F., and Blassingame, J.W. (1982). *Long Memory: The Black Experience In America.* New York: Oxford University Press.

Borsodi, R. (1965). "The Neglected Science of Values": Eight Propositions About Values." *Journal of Human Relations,* Vol. 13, pp. 433-445.

Boyd-Franklin, N. (1989). *Black Families in Therapy.* New York: The Guilford Press.

Brislin, R. (1993). *Understanding Culture's Influences on Behavior.* Fort Worth, Texas: Harcourt Brace Javanovich College Publishers.

Chandler, C. K., J. M. Holden and C. A. Kolander (1992). "Counseling for Spiritual Wellness: Theory and Practice," *Journal of Counseling and Development,* November/December, Vol. 71, pp. 168ff.

Cook, N. D. and S. Kono (1977). "Black Psychology: The Third Great Tradition." *The Journal of Black Psychology,* Vol. 3, No. 2, pp. 18-28.

Dancy, Jr. Joseph (1977). *The Black Elderly: A Guide for Practitioners.* Ann Arbor, Michigan: The University of Michigan Press.

Devore, N., and Schlesinger, E. G. (1991). *Ethnic-Sensitive Social Work Practice.* New York: Macmillan, Third Edition.

Frankl, V. (1978). *The Unheard Cry for Meaning: Psychotherapy and Humanism.* New York, N.Y.: Simon and Schuster.

Greene, R. R. (1986). *Social Work with the Aged and Their Families.* New York: Aldine de Gruyter.

Harel, Z. McKinney, E. A., Williams, M. (Eds.), (1990). *The Black Aged.* Newbury Park, CA: Sage Publications.

Hayles, Robert, V., Jr. (1991). "African Americans Strengths: A Survey of Empirical Findings." In Reginald R. Jones (ed.), *Black Psychology,* 3rd ed. Berkeley, California: Cobb and Henry Publishers.

Heisel, M. A., Faulkner, A. O. (1982). "Religiosity in an Older Black Population." *Gerontologist,* 22, No. 4.

Heriot, C. S. (1992). "Spirituality and Aging." *Holistic Nursing Practice,* Vol. 7, No. 1, pp. 22-31. Aspen Publications.

Hill, R. B. (1972). *The Strengths of Black Families.* New York, New York: National Urban League.

Howard, G. (1991). "Culture Tales: A Narrative Approach to Thinking, Cross-Cultural Psychology and Psychotherapy." *American Psychologist,* Vol. 46, pp. 187-197.

Jackson, J. J. (1971). "Black Grandparents: Who Needs Them?" In *The Black Family.* Belmont, California: Wadsworth Company.

Jones, R. L. (1991). *Black Psychology.* Third Edition, Berkley, CA: Cobb and Henry Publishers.

Kart, C. S. (1994). *The Realities of Aging.* Boston, Mass.: Allyn & Bacon.

Kluckhohn, C. (1951). "Values and Value Orientations." In Talcott Parsons and Edward A. Shils, eds., *Toward Theory of Action.* Cambridge, Massachusetts: Harvard University Press.

Koenig, H. G., Kvale, J. N., and Ferrel, G. (1988). "Religion and Well-Being in Later Life." *Gerontologist,* 28, No. 1.

Knox, D. J. (1985). "Spirituality: A Tool in the Assessment and Treatment of Black Alcoholics and Their Families." *Alcoholism Treatment Quarterly,* 2, No. 3/4, pp. 31-44.

Logan, S. M. L., Freeman, E. M., McRoy, R. G. (1990). *Social Work Practice With Black Families*. White Plains, N.Y.: Longman.

Martin, Elmer and JoAnne Mitchell Martin (1979). 'Problems of Urban Life." In *The Black Extended Family*. Chicago: The University of Chicago Press, pp. 83-93.

Maslow, A. (1971). *Farther Reaches of Human Nature*. New York: Viking Press.

Mbiti, J. S. (1969). *African Religions and Philosophies*. Garden City, New York: Anchor Books.

Mitchell H. and N. Lewter (1986). *Soul Theology: The Heart of American Black Culture*. San Francisco: Harper & Row.

Moberg, D. O. (1971). "Spiritual Well-Being." *White House Conference on Aging*. Washington, D.C., Background Paper.

Moberg, D. O. (1970). "Religion in the Later Years." In A.M. Hoffman (Ed.), *The Daily Needs and Interests of Older Persons*. Springfield, IL: Charles C Thomas.

Neugarten, B., and K. Weinstein (1964). "The Changing American Grandparents." *Journal of Marriage and the Family*, Vol. 26, No. 2, pp. 199-204.

Nobles, W. (1980). "African Philosophy: Foundations for Black Psychology." In R. Jones (Ed.), *Black Psychology* (2nd ed.). New York: Harper & Row, pp. 23-36.

Nobles, W., L. Goddard, W. Cavil and Geage. (1987). *African American Families: Issues, Insights and Directions*.

O'Driscoll, M. P. (1976). "Value and Culture Contact: Some Perspective and Problems." In Richard Brislin, ed., *Topics in Culture Learning*, Vol. 4, pp. 8-9. Honolulu: East-West Center.

Philibert, M. (1981). "The Phenomenological Approach to Images of Aging." In LeFeore, C. LeFeore, P. (eds.) *Aging and The Human Spirit: A Reader in Religion and Gerontology*, 2nd ed. Chicago, Illinois: Exploration Press.

Ross, P. (1981). "Discovering the Spiritual Resources in Aging." In LeFeore, C. LeFeore, P. (eds.) *Aging and the Human Spirit: A Reader in Religion and Gerontology*, 2nd ed. Chicago, Illinois: Exploration Press.

Sperry, R. W. (1974). "Science and the Problem of Values." *Zygon*, Vol 9, pp. 7-21.

Staples, R. (1986). *The Black Family*. Belmont, CA: Wadsworth.

Taylor, R. J., (1986). "Religious Participation Among Elderly Blacks." *Gerontologist*, 26, 637-642.

Thurman, H. (1979). *With Head and Heart*. New York, N.Y.: Hartcourt Brace Javanovich.

Thurman, H. (1963). *Disciplines of the Spirit*. Richmond, Indiana: Friends United Press.

White, J. (1984). *The Psychology of Blacks: An Afro-American Perspective*. Englewood Cliffs, N.J.: Prentice Hall.

Wilson, Emily H. (1983). *Hope and Dignity: Older Black Women of the South*. Philadelphia: Temple University Press.